CARDIOLOGY FOR WOMEN

Cardiology for Women

Dr Jerzy George Dyczynski

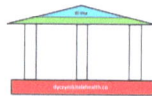

Contents

IV |

This book is dedicated to all women, their genius, bravery, and compassion. Spiritually, this book is dedicated to the heart of the Holy Mary.

You should seek advice from a qualified healthcare professional

Information in this book is intended as general summary information that is made available to the public. It is not intended to provide specific medical advice, or to take the place of a qualified healthcare professional. Information resources are designed to help readers to better understand their own health and diagnosed conditions. You are urged to consult with qualified health care providers for diagnosis and treatment and for answers to personal health care questions.

1

Introduction

He heals the brokenhearted and binds up their wounds. Psalm 147. Verse 3.

You may be surprised to learn that most of the heart and cardiovascular research on major topics in Cardiology, including Angina pectoris and heart attack, has been performed on male populations.

Women's hearts, distinct in size, structure, function, and emotion processing, face unique challenges in cardiovascular health. The term Angina pectoris, derived from the Latin 'angere' and 'pectus' translates to a strangling feeling in the chest, describing the symptom of coronary artery narrowing.

Women, with their bodies designed for beauty, comfort, and acts of charity, are more susceptible to pain than men due to the presence of internal reproductive female organs and feminine hormones.

Angina pectoris can manifest uniquely in women, including in the lower abdomen. You can feel pain, pressure, tightness, or discomfort in the lower abdomen. Muscle tension in the pelvic area can activate the pelvic stress reflex, causing pain and discomfort even in the uterus.

The pelvic stress reflex can strongly influence your breathing, and pelvic pain contributes to raising distress levels, underscoring the need to address stress urgently. The pain may radiate to your lower back, hips, or thighs, worsening with exertion or stress and improving with rest, a key diagnostic feature. This makes it more challenging for you as a woman to manage stress and maintain integrity under stressful circumstances.

Women are known for their warmth, tenderness in the heart, and love, which they express through affectionate gestures. These unique characteristics have significantly influenced the development of Cardiology for women, as their hearts in distress unfold and progress differently than in men.

Experiencing a "broken heart" due to emotional trauma, such as the loss of a loved one or an unexpected life event, maybe more than just a figure of speech. A broken heart is an existing medical condition known as stress cardiomyopathy. Heart distress occurs mainly in women because they are more sensitive and tend to have smaller, more delicate hearts and thinner coronary arteries. While it can occasionally affect men, over 90% of the situations where the heart is in extreme distress occur in women.

Recent research has shown that intense emotional stress, which you can experience multiple times during your lifespan, can trigger the release of stress hormones that cause multiple spasms in the coronary arteries and temporarily weaken your heart, leading to symptoms resembling those of a heart attack. Your distressed heart in this situation is exposed to cardiovascular and metabolic stress.

Cardiovascular stress is the impact of a stressed brain on the heart and blood vessels. Increased heart rate and high blood pressure contribute to developing your distressed heart. It triggers the release of hormones like Adrenaline, which can cause a further surge in heart rate and blood pressure. Excessive stress can produce coronary artery spasms and reduce the blood flow to your heart muscle. Cardiovascular stress also causes electrical instability, disrupting the heart's electrical system and leading to irregular heartbeats or palpitations. Your distressed heart demands more oxygen to overcome this unusual situation.

Metabolic stress is caused by your body's low energy levels during an intense stress reaction. It slows down the biochemical reactions and energy production. This leads to disruption of your metabolic wheel. Metabolic stress affects your cellular breathing negatively. Low cellular breathing produces an inflammatory response and hormonal imbalance and can result in tissue damage. Metabolic stress manifests when your body needs more energy than it currently has. Sometimes, it feels like chronic fatigue.

Women experiencing distressed hearts, also known as stress cardiomyopathy, may display symptoms that very closely mimic a heart attack resulting from the spasming of two or even more major coronary arteries supplying essential parts of their heart muscle.

Like everything else, your body comprises vibrating and continuously charged atoms and sub-atomic particles. This electromagnetic reality is not a one-time event but a continuous process, a constant reminder for you to be aware of the electromagnetic nature of your own body when considering your heart in distress.

To visualize the electromagnetic reality of the heart and body, a Dutch physician, Dr. Willem Einthoven, invented an electrocardiogram, or ECG in abbreviation. An ECG is a visual representation of this electromagnetic activity. The picture displays a registration of an ECG by a female athlete on the left and a diagram of a single, perfect heartbeat on the right.

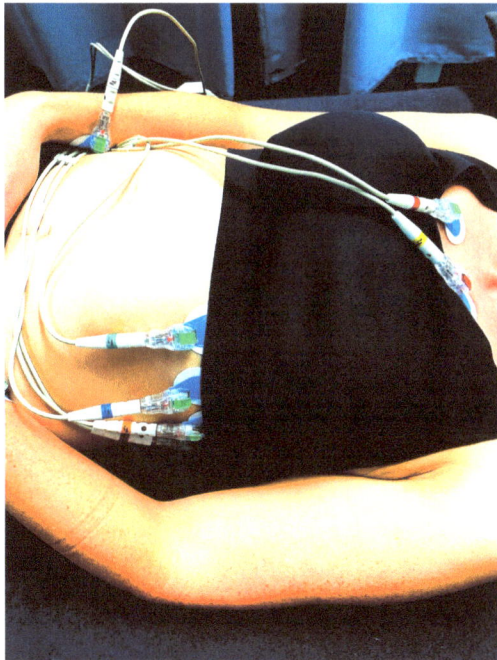

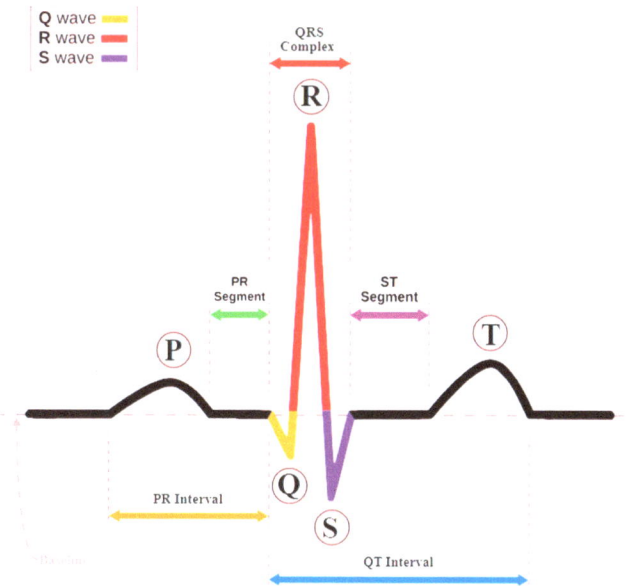

Picture 1. A screening ECG being performed in a female athlete. Johnorchard - Own work on the left. Diagram of a single heartbeat as seen on ECG. Created by Agateller (Anthony Atkielski) on the right. Wikipedia.

ECG is the most widely used tool for diagnosing distressed hearts. It registers the electromagnetic waves of the heart around the baseline.

The constant spin of hydrogen protons generates electricity that flows through your body. The atoms and subatomic particles of your heart cells vibrate at a specific electromagnetic frequency, which forms the unique signature of your "quantum body." These electric signals travel throughout your body and can be read and registered. Your signature pattern will then appear during your ECG registration. The electrical current, primarily produced by your heart, is the expression of life.

The ECG consists of the QRS complex, which captures the heart's excitation and contraction. At the same time, the T wave illustrates the heart's relaxation.

Imagine that only one heartbeat features more than ten elements and represents just a single perfect heartbeat. The standard ECG captures hundreds of heartbeats from 12 different channels in a typically recorded ECG reading.

Each individual's ECG reading is unique, and countless variations of normality and abnormalities exist. Therefore, computerized assessment is crucial in aiding doctors in understanding and interpreting these readings.

The ECG is a medical assessment tool that recognizes a threatening heart attack or a heart in distress. Your ECG result is then meticulously reviewed by a skilled doctor, who draws conclusions about your heart condition. The doctor ensures that you receive all information and that you understand its meaning correctly.

The arrival of modern ECG machines and computerized assessment systems has revolutionized this process, providing valuable support to doctors and significantly enhancing the accuracy of their conclusions during ECG examinations.

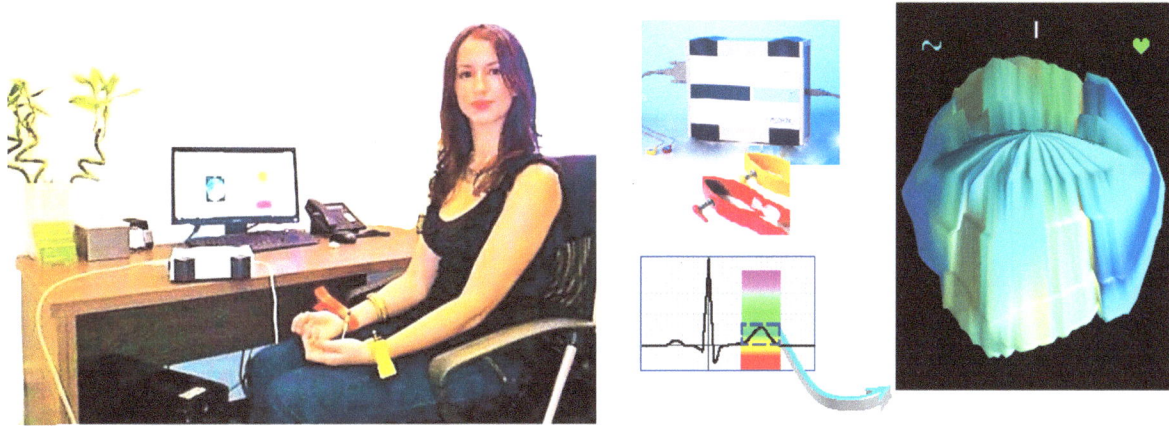

Picture 2. Registration of a normal ECG. Courtesy Amelia.

A small device connected to your body with clamps on the hands and ankles captures the heart's electromagnetic field, a scientific term for the electrical activity produced by the heart. This captured data is projected as the heart's portrait on a computer screen. This modern ECG heart screening technique uses clear visuals that allow you to understand what happened to your heart effectively. One picture has more information than one thousand words.

When you see your ECG individual pattern, you can immediately understand your heart health. An ECG is a noninvasive test that is simple and painless and helps assess many heart conditions, including abnormal heart rhythm, palpitations, distressed heart, coronary artery spasms, heart attack, heart wall thickness, electrical blocks, and heart damage.

Some modern electrocardiogram (ECG) devices provide a color-coded representation of the ECG for all recorded channels, your pattern of the heart and cardiovascular system, also known as the color-coded pattern or a cardio portrait. This device captures the heart's electromagnetic field accurately and in real-time, ensuring that you and your doctors are always up to date with your heart's condition. It is an excellent technique for visualizing your heart in distress and making it understandable for you.

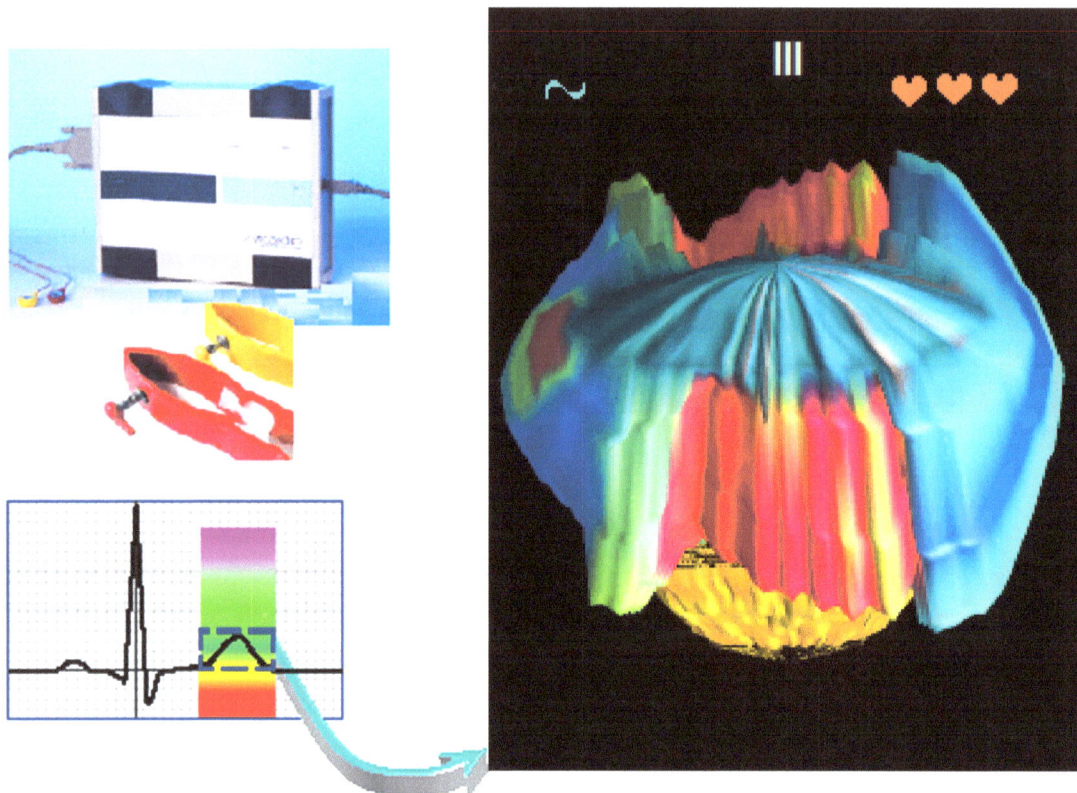

Picture 3. This is an ECG registration. It shows a broken ECG pattern of the highly distressed heart of a young woman.

This ECG registration belonged to a young woman. The man she fell in love with has broken her heart, and she was deeply disappointed with the relationship. After three weeks of intense treatment, including a consultation with a cardiologist, weekly acupuncture treatment, naturopathic consultations, and psychological counseling, the following pattern of her ECG registration was obtained.

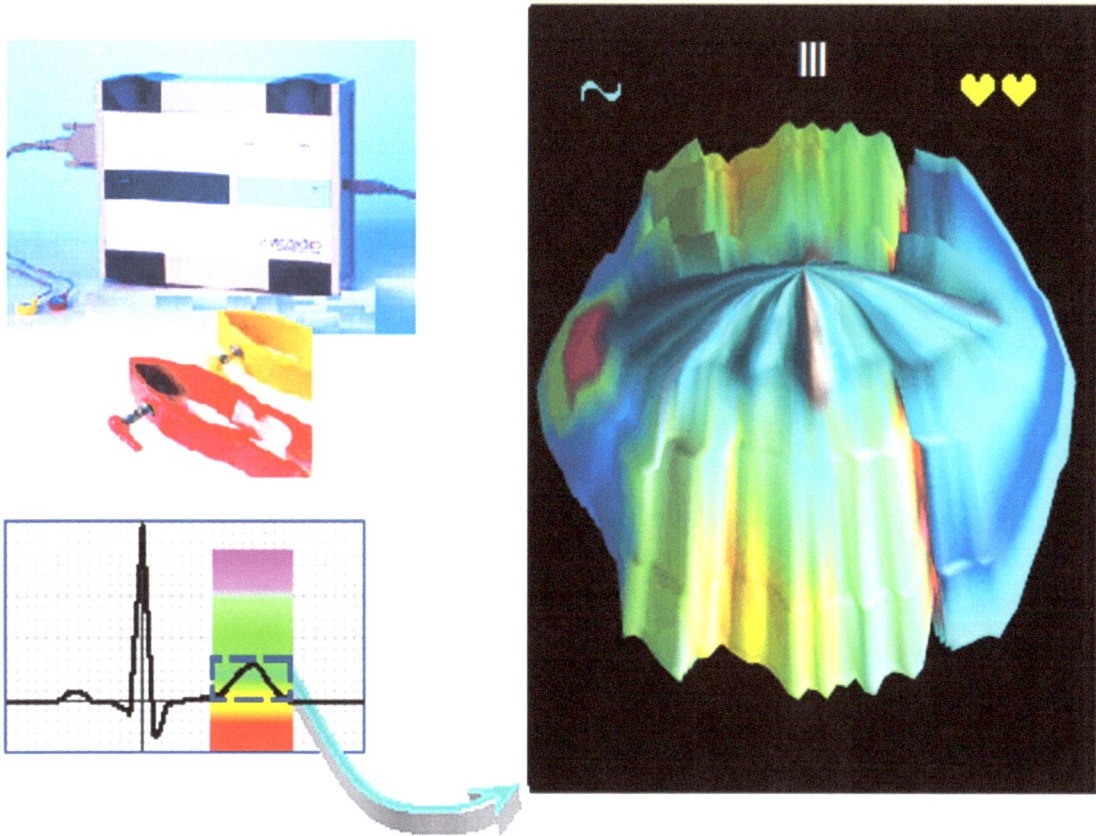

Picture 4. This is a follow-up registration of the ECG of the same young woman. The ECG indicates that the healing process is in progress. She was recovering from her once-broken heart pattern.

2

Your beautiful heart

Your adornment must not be merely the external—braiding the hair, wearing gold jewelry, or putting on apparel; but it should be the hidden person of the heart, with the imperishable quality of a gentle and quiet spirit, which is precious in the sight of God. 1 Peter, Verse 3-4.

Please realize that your heart is your best friend. It is at the core of your bodily functions and it determines your health, mobility, vitality, and intellectual wellness. Your intelligent heart performs its functions properly only with sufficient oxygen. Consider your heart and its language as the compass that guides your actions.

Your heart has an energy channel that connects to your brain, solar and pelvic plexus, internal organs, and muscles. This channel, starting in the heart and ending at the small finger on both sides of your body. Every intention that originates in your heart is manifested and performed through your hands, underscoring the heart's influence on your daily activities.

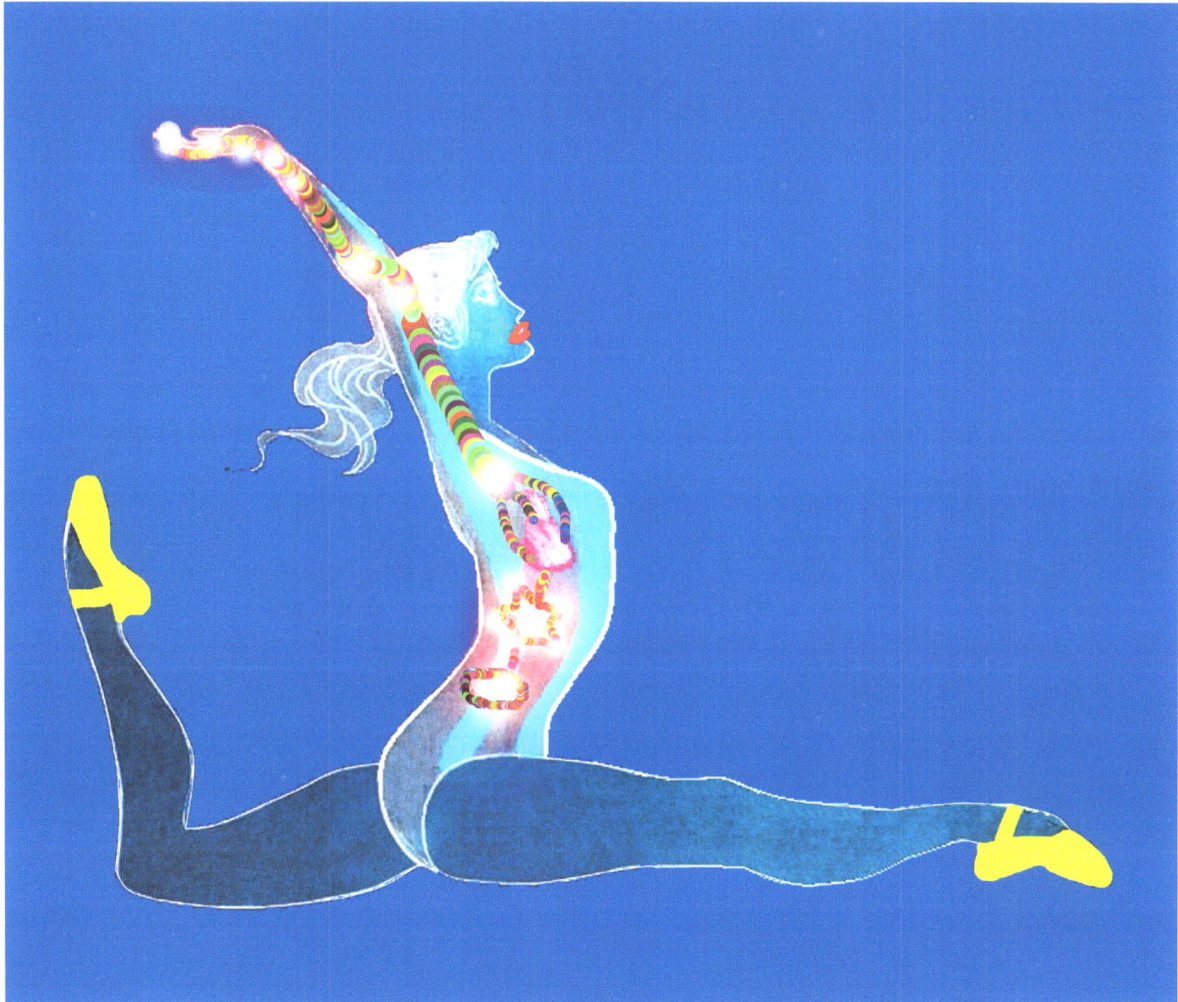

Picture 5. Heart energy channel and its connection to the solar and pelvic plexus.

Your feelings, thoughts, desires, and actions are linked to your heart and your brain. They build the intangible aspects of your spiritual existence. Your heart-brain intimate relationship governs your emotions and intentions, influencing your external expressions and intellect. Your ability to experience peaceful rest, sound sleep, blissful relaxation moments, and coordinated movements depends on the health of your heart and brain.

Take solace in your heart. It is a tireless, dedicated, and empathetic organ. It has a unique space where love, trust, justice, wisdom, and grace come together. During quiet moments or meditation, your heart actively connects you with the fabric of the Universe, allowing you to experience a sense of oneness, sometimes even a state of bliss. Many spiritually attuned nuns, monks, athletes, yoga instructors, and renowned yogis have encountered this extraordinary unity. It is a unique blend of positive emotions such as love, compassion, joy, calmness, contentment, and serenity, all acting in harmony at once.

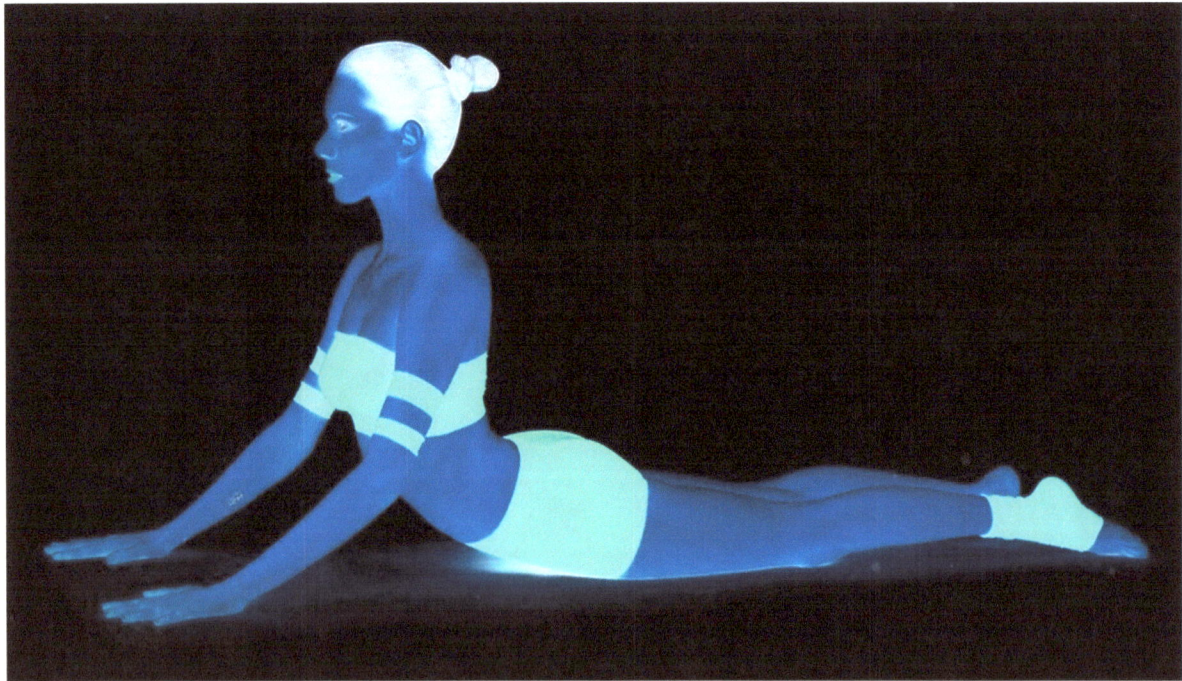

Picture 6. Nina Mel, a prominent yoga teacher by Kennguru Wikipedia. Inverse colors.

This extraordinary state of bliss is familiar to anyone who has ever been in love. You, too, have experienced a moment of this universal unity—where body, soul, mind, heart, and spirit align in unprecedented perfection. Such transformative moments stay with you for a lifetime. When you recall them, they act as a catalyst that elevates you to your highest potential and inspires you to push your performance beyond your limits.

Your heart is always in motion; it never rests. It tirelessly pumps oxygenated, fresh blood to your brain when you are intellectually active or to your muscles during physical activities, adjusting its pace and volume based on your body's needs. This relentless dedication is not just a physical feat but a source of inspiration and motivation to strive for the best version of yourself.

Your heart is amazing at its work. It is an organ that distinguishes between healthy and unhealthy tendencies in your body and environment. Its inherent intelligence is always present and meticulously tuned, encouraging you to explore the complexity of your own body.

3

Your perfect heart

And give my son Solomon a perfect heart to keep Your commandments, Your testimonies, and Your statutes, and to do them all, and to build the temple for which I have made provision. 1 Chronicles 29:19.

Your very special heart is equipped with a built-in array of mechanical bio-sensors that detect signals related to blood circulation, ensuring its smooth flow. These sensors, known as receptors, are strategically located in your blood vessels and the heart's internal walls. They instantly identify any irregular flow within your heart's four chambers and monitor vital factors like oxygen saturation, water content, minerals in the blood, and blood pressure.

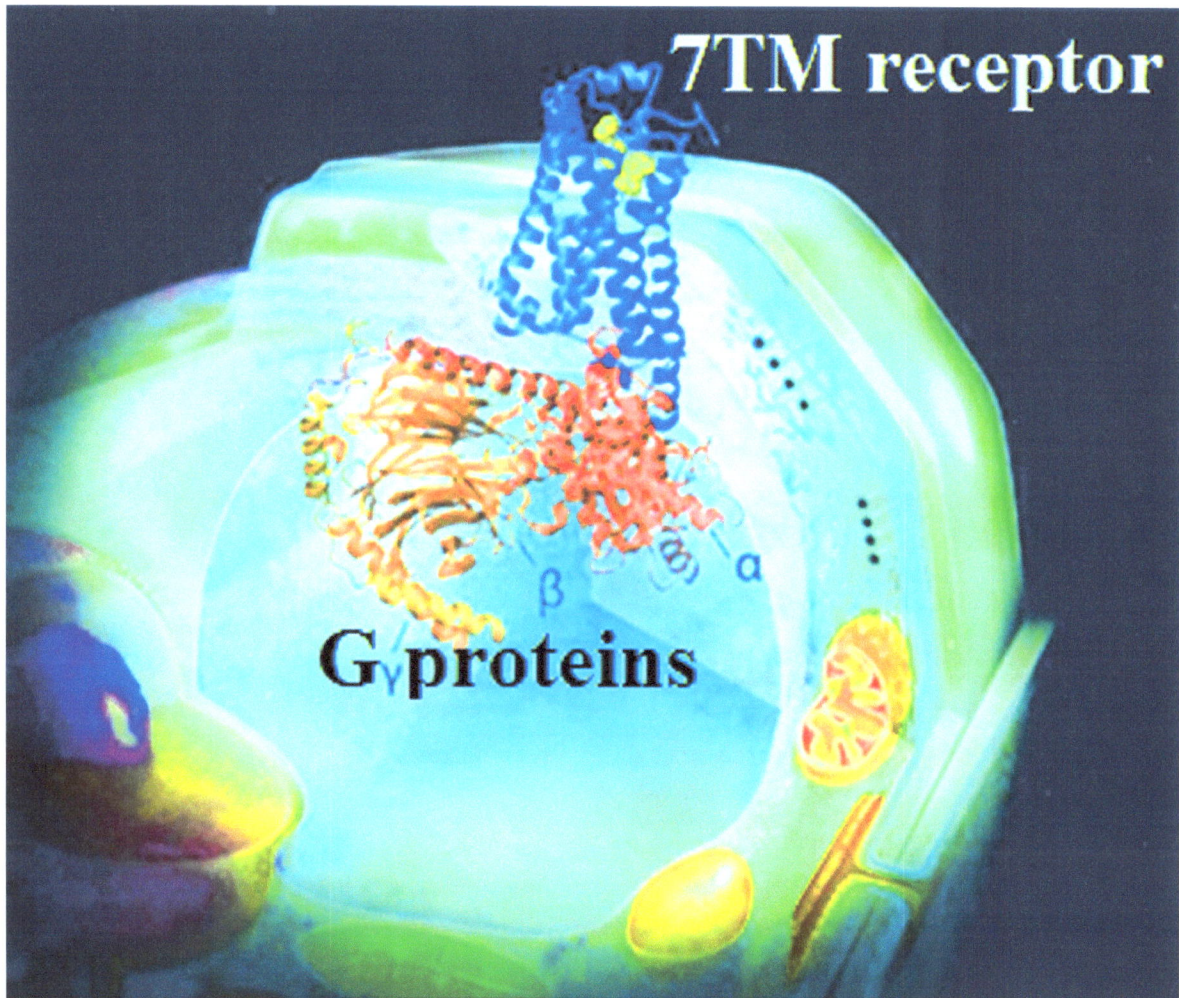

Picture 7. The biosensor is abundant in every cell of your body. Two mini-crystals of cholesterol at the top of the 7 TM biosensor are marked with yellow color.

The heart, a dynamic and active organ, is connected to the body's interior and external environment via special 7TM bio-sensors. They span the cell membrane seven times. Like cellular smartphones, these bio-sensors are recipients and active senders of signals and messages. They are part of a larger system that includes your heart, brain, and DNA. When they encounter specific hormones, temperature changes, and mechanical influences, they report all imbalances, ensuring the entire system is in sync. These cellular bio-sensors detect vortex waves, high blood pressure, and scrambled vibrations caused by abnormal heartbeats. All these factors trigger the release of Adrenaline, a key player in the body's fight-or-flight response. Simultaneously, they kick-start the production of the protective heart hormones, ensuring your heart's well-being.

The 7 blades of the 7TM biosensor navigate the complex cell functions in all your heart's cells, showcasing the wonderful nature of your cardiac biology. Each biosensor contains two mini-crystals of cholesterol, positioned at the top and marked yellow. These crystals resonate with incoming and outgoing impulses and frequencies, adding a layer of complexity to the heart's cellular communication.

Cholesterol crystals are important for heart-brain communication, making cholesterol crucial for brain health. Every cell of your heart muscle is equipped with hundreds or more of these tiny biosensors and antennas, further highlighting your heart's marvelous nature.

The biosensors measure the volume and temperature of circulating blood and adjust them based on your body's immediate needs. Additionally, they sense pH balance and monitor mineral levels. When disturbances occur, these receptors diligently signal the release of specific heart hormones from your heart to restore your balance and equilibrium.

The heart's hormones are your body's guardians. The action of your four heart hormones is to protect balance and counteract stress, ensuring that your body stays calm. Type A is the first hormone identified as originating from the heart and managing the water household. Type B was discovered initially in the brain and is essential for its protection. These are just two examples of these protective hormonal heart agents.

Meet the two more members of your heart's hormone family. Type C, a key player in fostering regeneration, was first discovered in salmon. It is well known that fish, especially salmon, is good for your heart health. Type D shares similarities with the substance that disrupts the blood's clotting in the green mamba snake venom. This heart hormone regulates the blood clotting.

As you know now, your heart hormones' actions extend far beyond mere metabolism and energy production. They protect your heart and the integrity of your overall body health, influencing critical aspects of the stress response, fat metabolism, blood acidity/alkalinity, blood clotting, tissue oxygenation, and balance of your bodily water and minerals.

4

Your heart, the guardian of your health

*A*bove all else, guard your heart, for it is the wellspring of life. Proverbs 4:23.

Your heart strives for perfection in every moment. It can skillfully re-balance turbulent flow, the swirling motion of blood caused by a temporarily rigid heart wall due to a poor supply of fresh blood and low oxygenation.

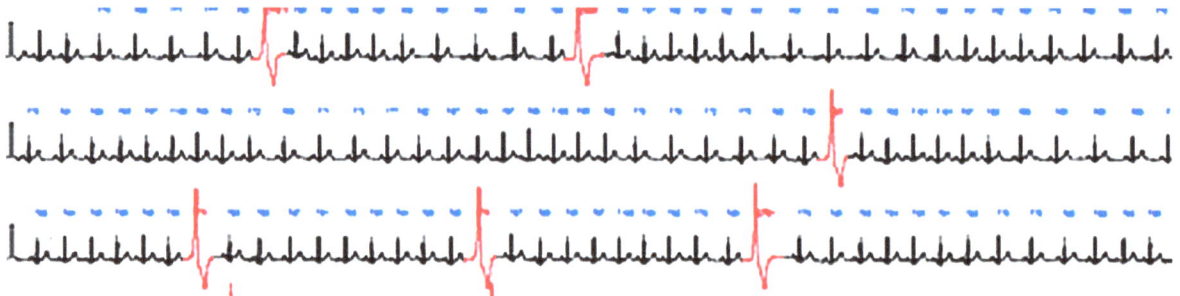

Picture 8. Abnormal heart beats marked with red color.

It can prevent premature ventricular beats that can disrupt smooth blood flow. Your heart maintains a steady rhythm, gently pulsating throughout your body. With astounding endurance,

16

it can generate a regular heartbeat without fail for 90 to 100 years, a remarkable feat of resilience. Each mechanical heartbeat produces an electrical-evoked potential in your brain, running through the spine and nervous system to every corner of your body. This constant stream of information reaches your cells, activating their sensors and ultimately influencing your DNA.

But your heart is more than just a physical organ; it opens in your emotions. This vital organ houses messenger RNA (mRNA) molecules that stimulate the production of hormones related to your feelings. These hormones, such as oxytocin and dopamine, are essential in regulating the intensity of your emotional responses. The dynamic flow of information is a vibrant cascade of living signals. It renews itself with each heartbeat.

Acknowledge the incredible power of your heart. It is not only essential for your survival but is also intimately connected to your emotional well-being. Embrace your heart and cherish every one of your heartbeats.

Thanks to its continuous capacity for renewal, your heart beats tirelessly for over 90 to 100 years. In 2010, Harvard University in the USA unveiled a groundbreaking revelation: your heart is perpetually generating adult omnipotent stem cells. This discovery marks a turning point in regenerative medicine, illuminating a path of hope for medical innovations. The heart's regenerative potential is a reason for optimism and hope for the future of medical science.

The 2012 Nobel Prize was awarded to John B. Gurdon and Dr. Shinya Yamanaka for their pioneering work reprogramming mature cells into omnipotent adult stem cells for all human organs. Organs such as the liver, kidney, and spleen's capacity to generate adult omnipotent stem cells are vital for the body's ability to renew throughout life.

This research confirmed that even organs with slower regenerative rates, like your heart, which requires approximately 20 years for complete renewal, and your brain, which needs around 40 years to replace all its neurons and nerve cells, can heal and regenerate effectively.

Is it not amazing? You can create four or even five hearts in your life and build two to three brains from scratch over your lifetime. This is your visionary reality that your heart is the leading force in your body's self-organizing system.

The beautiful description of the adult stem cell can be found in the book *Life and Teachings of the Masters of the Far East* by Baird Spalding, published in 1991:

"As the cell divides and creates a new cell, our thought is implanted upon it... In the first cell, all is perfect. That cell was first known as the "Christ cell" or anointed cell. It is always just as young as ever it was. It never takes on old age. It is the primal spark of life. The body responds when we implant our thoughts of limitation, old age, or any condition outside of perfection. Cells born from the first cell take on its image. Originally, it was the image and likeness of God. It is perfect in every way. But it becomes the form we carry in our minds...if we always carry the image of perfection, what will it do for these cells? It will build perfection." (Vol. 6, Page 78)

5

The genius of the woman's heart

In Nature you behold the mother aspect of God, full of beauty, gentleness, tenderness, and kindness.
Paramahansa Yogananda.

Saint John Paul II had profound respect and admiration for women, as is evident in his eloquent descriptions of their genius and dignity. In 1995, as a Pope in the Vatican, he wrote the "Letter to Women," where he articulated the qualities of feminine genius. He stated that women have a unique love for others, prioritizing humans above all else and recognizing the greatness of each individual soul.

Saint John Paul II foresaw the increasing role of women in addressing and solving serious societal problems. He believed that a greater presence of women would be invaluable in society. It will challenge the existing male-dominated systems, prompting them to be redesigned in favor of a 'civilization of love.' This vision empowered women, highlighting their potential to shape a more compassionate and just society.

Another artistic inspiration for women's genius is the canvas created in Paris, France. It displays the great spirituality of post-Civil War America. This masterpiece from the 19th century, painted by the highly esteemed French painter Adolphe Yvon in Paris, is a symbolic procession that exalts the nation's glory, which women lead.

The Lady Republic's majestic white attire is at the heart of this procession. The Roman goddess Minerva, draped in her regal white and green robes, represents music, poetry, medicine, wisdom, commerce, weaving, and crafts, embodying the essence of wisdom and knowledge. Both stand atop a chariot drawn by lions, a sight that evokes a profound sense of awe and reverence. Leading the chariot are women, each representing a state, from New York to Illinois to Virginia, symbolizing this new time of American unity and its nation's incredible spiritual diversity.

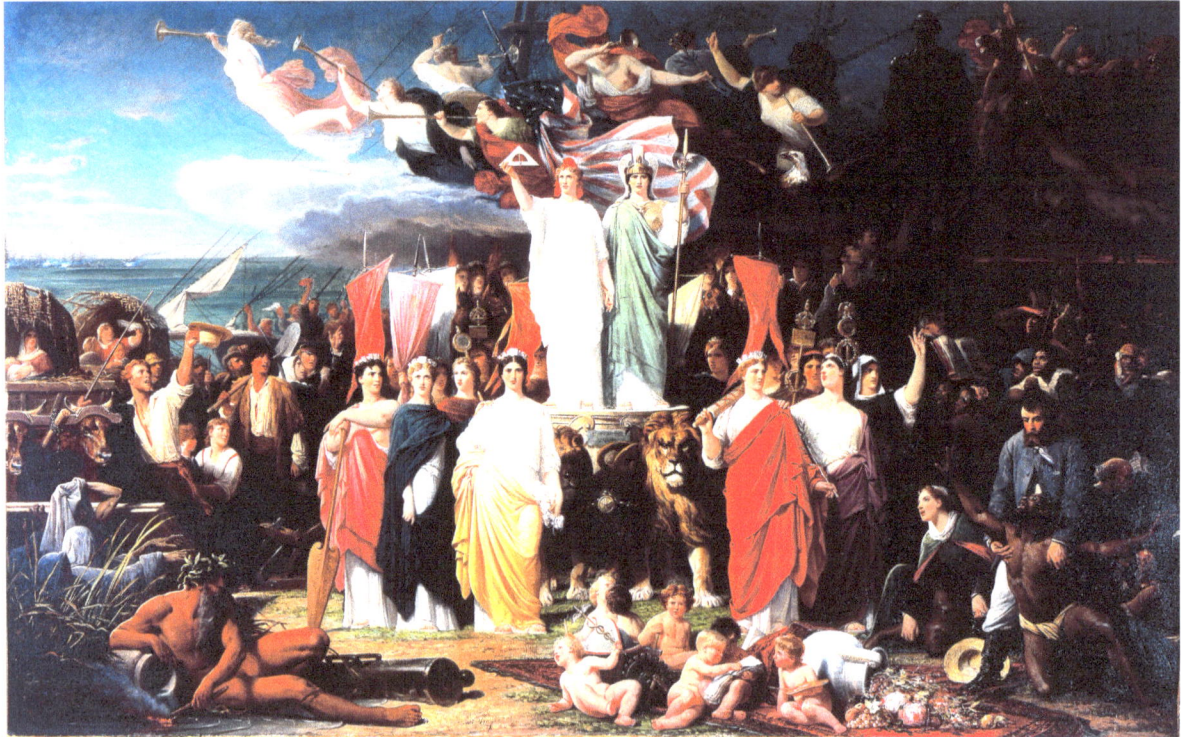

Picture 9. Genius of America. By Adolphe Yvon, Wikipedia.

According to St John Paul II, the "Genius of the woman's heart" refers to women's unique strengths and qualities, which make the world more human. The uniqueness of the feminine heart includes:

Exceptional receptivity: An active openness to receiving the gifts of life and love.

Great sensitivity: The ability to understand the deeper needs of the human heart and respond with love.

Magnificent generosity: A spirit of generosity that values the humanity in every person.

Maternity: The unique capacity for motherhood, both physical and spiritual, a nurturing force that brings warmth and care to the world.

Saint John Paul II emphasized and firmly believed that women's 'feminine genius' is vital to creating a culture of life and love. He also believed in and valued women's moral and spiritual strength. This unique and powerful force empowers and uplifts all humanity. This strength is deeply connected to their understanding that God entrusts the care of human beings to them in a unique and special way, making them integral to the divine order.

These qualities truly distinguish a woman's heart. The unique nature of women's genius encapsulates an indispensable role in shaping human society, underscoring the significance of their contribution. A woman's heart is often likened to a profound ocean of secrets, a vast expanse that holds deep emotions, thoughts, and dreams. Just as the sea conceals its treasures beneath the waves, so does a woman's heart hide its mysteries, inviting every man to explore its depths, a journey that is both intriguing and curious.

Saint John Paul II held Mary, the Blessed Mother, in the highest regard, seeing her as the 'highest expression of the feminine genius.' This profound view of Mary as the source of feminine virtue and strength can inspire women to strive for similar greatness.

6

Feminine revolution

But the heavenly Jerusalem is the free woman, and she is our spiritual mother. Galatians Chapter 4, Verse 26.

The feminine revolution, the modern women's movement, is a powerful force that advocates for women's dignity, intelligence, and extraordinary human potential. It champions the right of women to make personal decisions about pregnancy and their professional development, empowering them to take control of their lives. The movement of feminine revolution emerged in a system of social structures and practices in which men dominated, oppressed, exploited, and coercively controlled women.

Men have been challenged to expand women's educational and career opportunities, and their concept of unequal pay was dismantled. The image of women as an unsatisfactory imitation or substitute for men in societal expectations is being redefined. The movement has stressed that women should not be passive and subordinate to men and that personal aspirations should be given equal importance to family.

The availability of "The Pill" had changed it. It became a medical lifeline to the freedom of modern women and was a seismic shift in various aspects of social life, including women's health, fertility trends, laws and policies, religion, interpersonal relationships, family roles, feminist issues, and their relations with men.

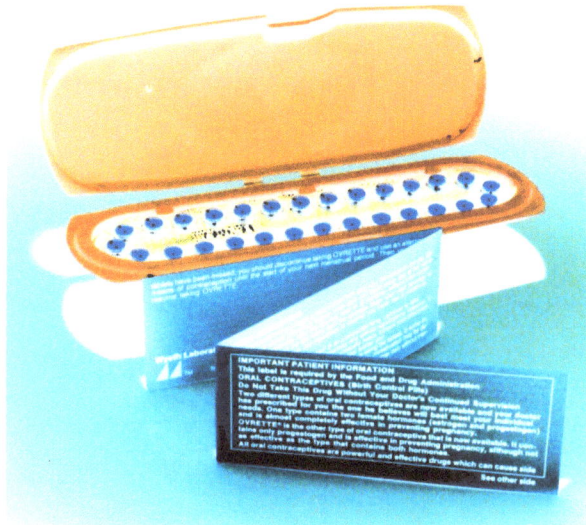

Picture 10. By The U.S. Food and Drug Administration - Patient Package Insert for Oral Contraceptives (FDA 079), Inverse color view. Public Domain,

2.7 billion or 70 percent of young women worldwide have used or now use a modern contraceptive method, demonstrating the global impact of this social movement. This is not just a personal choice, but a global movement that is shaping the future of women's health. The countries with the highest oral contraception rates are Finland, Switzerland, Canada, the United Kingdom, and China. This global reach underscores the importance of the pill as a symbol of freedom and its influence and significance in the feminine revolution.

The introduction of "The Pill" was a pivotal moment for women, allowing them to make choices about their lives, particularly in the workplace. It was a significant step towards women's liberation and autonomy.

However, it is important for you to be aware of the health risks associated with the pill, as this knowledge can empower you to make informed decisions about your heart health. The potential risks of oral, hormonal anti-conception, and hormone replacement therapy HRT. The irregular estrogenic profile and insufficient levels of progesterone are the hidden factors in the development of a distressed woman's heart, broken heart syndrome, and eventually heart attacks in women.

Taking estrogen and progesterone as birth control pills or in another form of hormone application than the pill can also cause an increase in blood clotting and high cholesterol levels and, in turn, can lead to a heart attack. Being informed about these risks can empower you to make informed decisions about your general and heart health.

Incredible results of contemporary research confirm that the contraceptive pill can change the thickness of the gray matter and amount of your brain neurons, particularly in areas important for regulating emotions.

In other words, the use of the pill could deeply affect your brain anatomy and functionality. The decline of the gray matter in the brain can be reversible, but it takes about a year to reverse it when you stop taking the pill. The resulting alteration of your brain function can cause anxiety.

The pill also reduces the number of endogenous sex hormones, which can lead to poor activation of estrogen bio-sensors, tensions in the pelvic area, including the uterus, and, more often, chronic pelvic pain.

Understanding the benefits of natural methods to prevent pregnancy can give you a sense of control and confidence, knowing that you are making informed and good choices about your body and heart health. Natural birth control and fertility awareness are methods that are not only reliable and effective, but they also inspire you to explore the knowledge and a deeper understanding of your body's natural rhythms. They do not involve devices or hormone manipulation to prevent pregnancy. Instead, you can track menstruation, cervical mucus, and basal temperature to predict ovulation.

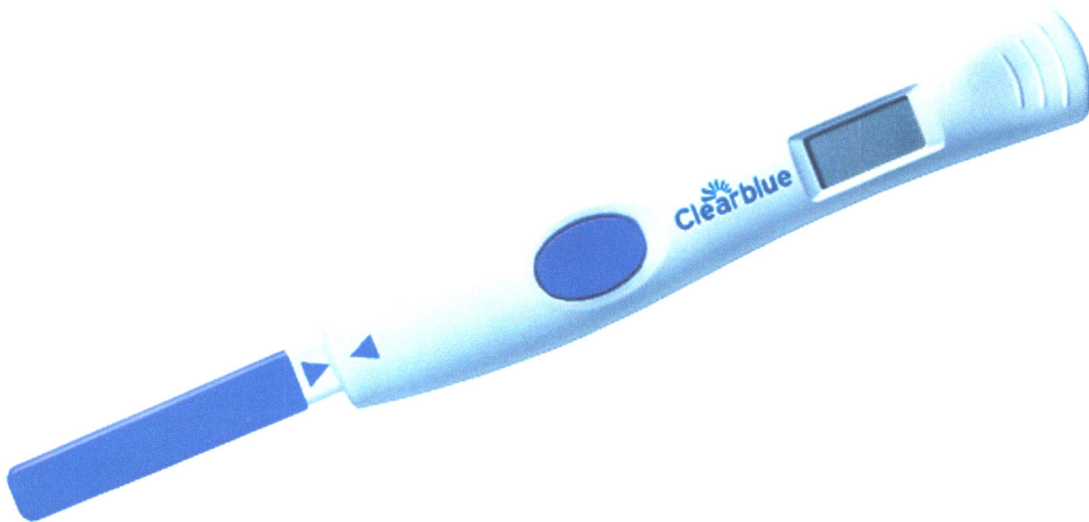

Picture 11. Clearblue Advanced Digital Ovulation Test. Wikipedia.

These simple and easy tests are not 100% accurate, but they are very close. Research suggests that ovulation tests have an accuracy of 99%. The natural methods are not only effective and practical but also reliable.

Your female hormones, estrogen and progesterone, protect your heart from the damaging effects of stress for about 20 to 25 years. However, as you reach the mid-30s and 40s, these hormone levels naturally decline, making you more vulnerable to the negative impacts of sudden stress. This decline, known in medical language as menopause can cause symptoms like hot flushes, night sweats, sleep disturbances and mood changes. It can be a moment for some women to consider hormone replacement therapy HRT.

It is important to be aware that taking progesterone with estrogen to compensate for the decline can potentially increase distress for your heart and even lead to a threatening heart attack.

The historical success of hormone replacement therapy (HRT) was based on the effective relief of unpleasant symptoms, particularly hot flushes and sweating, that often precede menopause. However, this success was not without its consequences, as the use of HRT has been linked later to the occurrence of distressed hearts, cancers, heart attacks, and strokes.

The book *Feminine Forever*, authored by American gynecologist Robert A. Wilson in 1966, significantly influenced the subculture and the lifestyle of women affected by menopause. Dr. Wilson's promotion of female hormone substitution therapy to treat menopause in all women led to a substantial increase in the use of hormone replacement therapy.

However, his assertions that female aging was a disease that could be cured with hormone substitution were later found to be incorrect. Dr Wilson did not realize that not only does the level of hormones change in the specific age of women, but the estrogen-related bio-sensors in the woman's body also undergo structural and functional alteration. The underlying process of estrogen biosensor loss and alterations, which follows natural changes and ends the fertility period, is an evidence to the body's natural processes. The effects of artificially added hormones do not reverse the alterations of estrogen biosensors but make them react adversely to added estrogens and progesterone.

Dr Wilson's historical misconceptions about hormone replacement therapy lacked strong research and evidence to support it. His assertions about estrogen and progesterone focused on only temporary benefits but went unchallenged for almost four decades until the Women's Health Initiative (WHI) study in 2002 in the USA.

The WHI, a monumental study involving over 160,000 women, contradicted Wilson's claims, demonstrating that HRT carries significant medical risks, such as heart attacks, strokes, breast cancer, and abnormal venous clots building. This study, on such a vast scale, clarified many misconceptions about the purported benefits of HRT.

The HRT study was initially designed to include a nine-year follow-up period. However, the preliminary report indicated an increased risk of breast cancer, coronary heart disease, stroke, and pulmonary embolism. As a result, the study had to be stopped earlier than planned for ethical reasons.

The broader discussion surrounding menopause underscores the belief that you have autonomy over your body and have the authority to make informed health decisions, including those related to HRT. This responsibility encourages you to take control of your health and to make the best choices, taking a proactive approach to your well-feeling.

In the years following the WHI, additional studies have shown a decrease in breast cancer rates among postmenopausal women. This significant decline is attributed to the reduction in the use of hormone replacement therapy. It offers hope, suggesting that effective menopause treatment can also be achieved through natural methods such as eating foods containing phytoestrogens and alternative techniques like medical acupuncture. This natural approach to symptoms of menopause can be an inspiration and encourage you to explore these natural therapy options.

Phytoestrogens are plant-based compounds that naturally mimic the effects of estrogen in the body. They can be found in diverse foods, from fruits and vegetables to legumes and grains, giving you various choices to incorporate into your diet.

Phytoestrogens are found in soy, lentils, legumes, flax seeds, cereal grains, and vegetables. The other phytoestrogens known as Coumestans were discovered in peas, beans, and clover sprouts. They also have anticancer effects.

Herbs like the Yarrow, Lady's mantle, and Horsetail taken as tea are excellent sources of phytoestrogens. These compounds can help alleviate menopause symptoms by naturally balancing your body's estrogen levels.

7

Prevention

For you, the Lord is a safe retreat; you have made the Most High your refuge. No disaster shall befall you, no calamity shall come upon your home. Psalm 91, Verse 10.

Stress is the body's natural and protective response to a physical or intellectual challenge. Your brain usually initiates stress cascade. It is a sign that your body is well equipped to handle difficult situations, but sometimes, your bodily stress symptoms tell you that you need to rest. There are two levels of your response to stress: cardiovascular and metabolic.

The symptoms of cardiovascular stress originate from your brain and heart and affect your entire body increasing the workload of your heart. It causes an accelerated heart rate and high blood pressure. Shallow breathing and low oxygenation are part of this response as your body prepares for a 'fight or flight' situation.

When you experience stress, the released Adrenaline makes your heart beat faster and work harder. It narrows your coronary blood vessels, leading to temporary spasms in your coronary arteries. These effects on your heart can cause Angina pectoris, lower jaw pain, and palpitations. They can manifest in your body as feminine manifestations. You can feel discomfort in your belly, pelvic region, and pelvic reflex with referred pain radiating to your hips, thighs, or even uterus.

At the same time, metabolic stress disrupts your normal balance, causing a nutrient scarce. The principal manifestation of your nutrient scarcity is a chronic lack of energy, sometimes known as chronic fatigue syndrome. It can also cause inflammation and tissue damage, underscoring the potential negative impact on your body and the profound weight of the long-lasting cardiovascular stress. Metabolic stress triggers the release of hormones that can lead to inflammatory responses in your body and affect your respiratory system, causing shortness of breath, shallow breathing, and poor oxygenation of your body.

Understanding metabolic stress can inspire you to take proactive steps to manage and mitigate your levels of Homocysteine, Vitamin B12, and Folate.

Applying orbital breathing and respiratory muscle training can help enormously. Using an oxygen concentrator can be a powerful tool for stress-counteracting actions. Gentle exercises, yoga, or spinal flow training can help restore the necessary metabolic balance. The inspired actions can also instill in you a sense of motivation and determination to commit more attention to your health and well-feeling.

Effectively managing your stress responses is a potent strategy to prevent your heart from experiencing distress. It can also mitigate the impact of long-acting cardiovascular stress on your major internal organs. Realizing that stress affects you at multiple levels can be daunting. Still, effective management can bring relief and hope for a healthier future.

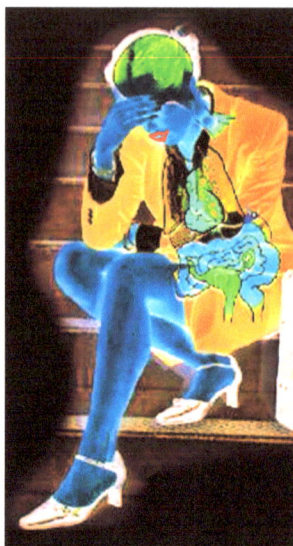

Picture 12. Stress affects your organs.

When distress strikes suddenly and unexpectedly, it often catches you off guard and is beyond your immediate control. A sudden surge of excessive Adrenaline in response to stress can overwhelm your heart muscle. This excess Adrenaline leads to the spasming and narrowing of your coronary arteries that supply your heart with fresh blood, significantly reducing blood flow to your heart.

When facing a distressing situation, remember that you hold the power of deep abdominal breathing. This simple yet effective technique can deactivate the released stress hormones, putting you in control of your body's response.

The left side of the diagram features an active molecule of Adrenaline. The unique gene COMT, the catechol-O-methyl-transferase, is a key player in the cardiovascular stress cascade. It can effectively silence the active Adrenaline. The 'O' in the COMT molecule originates from the oxygen in your body. The more oxygen in your body, the quicker it can help you de-stress. This insight, particularly the role of COMT and the role of your deep abdominal breathing in the process, will allow you to foster your de-stressing process.

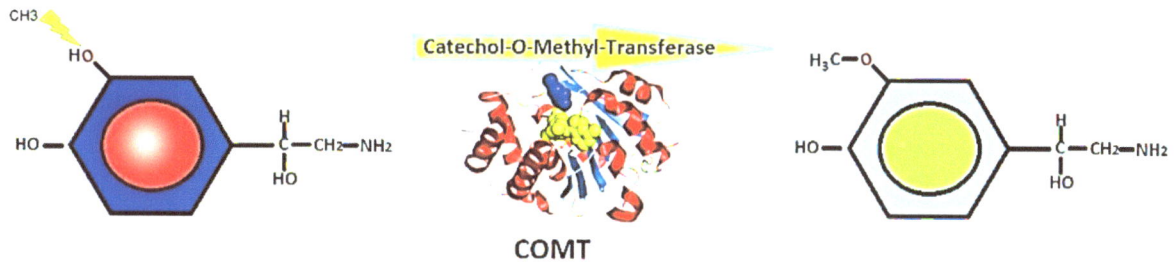

Picture 13. The diagram displays the deactivation of the stress hormones with oxygen.

1. Manage your stress effectively in your mind. The external factors, or outer situations, can often be the root cause of your stress. These could be anything from work deadlines to personal relationships. Get insight into what situations you can and cannot control.

2. Optimism can be cultivated by being cheerful and doing joyful, happy things every day you thought you could not do. This is a joy of achievement. If you have joy, you have everything.

3. Orbital breathing, a practice that includes deep and intentional breathing counteracts stress. It is your divine connection to the fabric of the Universe. In a moment of intense breathing, you can reach the holistic unity of your body and connect directly with your external environment. This experience can inspire you and show you that you can initiate this profound experience again. It will fill your life with more joy.

4. Consistent respiratory muscle training will give you further insights into your invisible components. It refers to the intangible aspects of your being, such as the heart, brain, mind, and soul, and how they are intensely entangled with your body and muscles. When your mind and soul are united, perfectly cooperating with your internal organs and muscles, it will create perfection in your body. When your heart, brain, mind, spirit, and body are in harmony, it gives peace and grace. Remember, the WHOLE is greater than the sum of its parts.

5. Be mindful of healthy nutrients. Plant-based nutrition is low in saturated fat and salt and high in fruits, vegetables, and whole grains, especially those not genetically modified, such as spelt or quinoa, which help prevent the buildup of coronary artery plaques and bring a relief to the metabolic stress.

6. Exercise whenever you can. Even several minutes of physical activity where you focus on your own body will support your heart health and accelerate your metabolism.

7. Schedule your sleep pattern correctly. Go to bed and wake up at the same time every day, allowing some exceptions on weekends. Wake up early with the sunlight. Rest when you need to. Ensure your bedroom is a sanctuary of tranquility. Spacious clean, dark, quiet, and cool bedroom provides the perfect environment for a restful night's sleep. It is important to train your brain to associate your bedroom with sleep only.

8. Be thankful for your medical team and enjoy your medical appointments, such as your GP, naturopath, reflexologist, osteopath, acupuncturist, or physio.

9. Embrace your meta-motivation, your soul's original impulses. As a self-actualized and updated woman, you are constantly striving to reach your full spiritual and intellectual potential. This is a conscious, continuous, intentional push for health and intellectual improvement, which drives your personal growth.

10. Make your daily Health Journal, a tool for personal growth and self-awareness. It will benefit you, help you de-stress, give you deeper insight into your internal processes, and help you better decode your body language and its interaction with your environment. It will also improve your self-awareness. Your journaling is the writing of your own story, a story of personal growth and self-awareness. Try to write in your journal every day, even if it is just a few minutes. Any place is right to write with or without interruptions. Be consistent and honest in your journaling, but remember, there is no right or wrong way. It is all about what works best for you. Forgive others or yourself to release negative feelings, and ask God or the higher genuine force of the Universe for forgiveness. As you change your mind, your behavior will change, and you will feel inspired and motivated by your personal development.

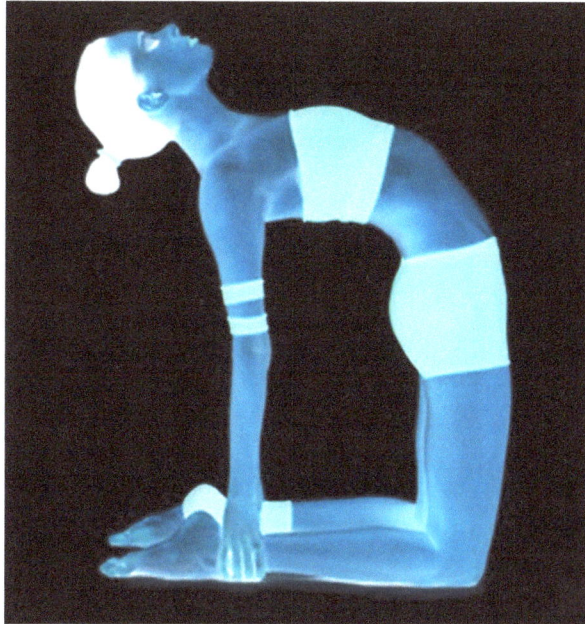

Picture 14 . Ultra-Asana by Nina-Mel. By Kennguru, Wikimedia. Inverse colors.

Your spiritual and physical progress is something to be proud of. Strive for grace in movements and for a spiritual gifts and blessings. Translating the grace of the Universe to a personal level is a spiritual quest. Achieving unity between the body, heart, mind, spirit, and soul is a profound mystery.

Again Jesus said, Peace be with you!... As the Father has sent me, I am sending you. And with that he breathed on them and said - receive the Holy Spirit. John 20:21-22

Your defining moment is the empowering decision to embark on daily respiratory muscle training. Regardless of your current health or activity level, this choice holds significant potential for you. Orbital breathing is not just a physical practice but also an intellectual one. It involves increasing self-awareness of your body's internal movements, such as the beating heart, pulse waves, and rhythmic breath movements.

Your respiratory muscle training RMT should be performed in a horizontal position at the beginning. When you start it, please lie down in a comfortable position. Put your hand on your tummy to control the movements of the diaphragm.

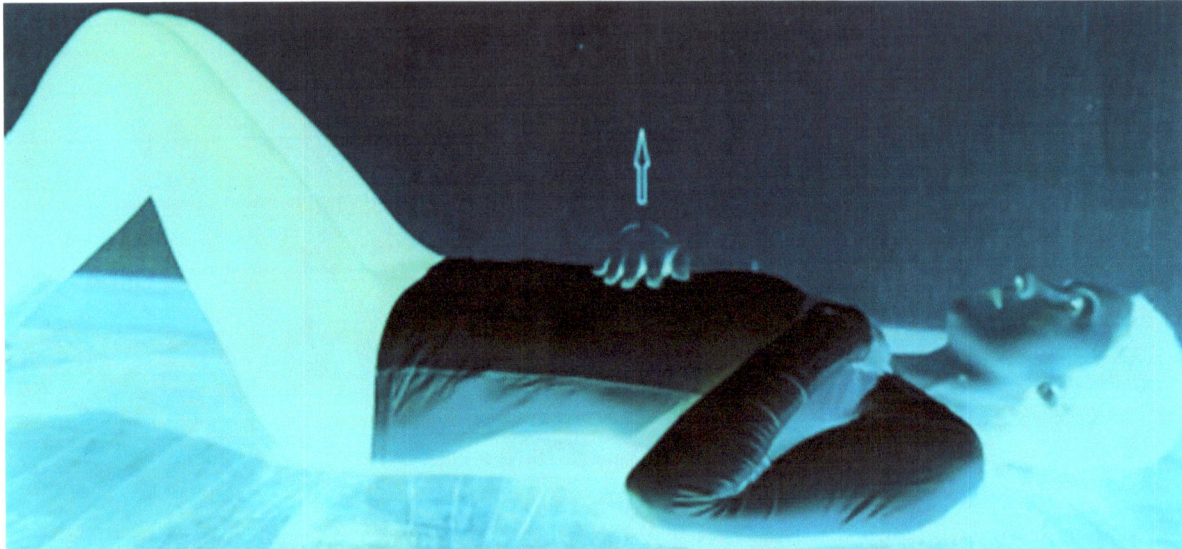

Picture 15. Abdominal breathing, Courtesy Brittany.

Diaphragmatic breathing is the most effective method for delivering increased oxygen and energy to the cells.

Here it is how:

1. Lie down somewhere comfortable and put your hand on your tummy.
2. Inhale – fill the lower part of your abdomen by diaphragmatic inhalation.
3. Keep inhaling – expand the middle section of the chest, increasing volume.
4. Even more – fill the upper chest and the top of the lungs, just below the collar bones to the brim.

5. Hold for about 3 seconds for increased oxygen ingestion. This little pause will maximize gas exchange in the lungs.

6. Then, wholly and forcefully exhale with a big "puff" or "whoosh."

Do this 5 to 10 times. It does not take long before you feel refreshed and energized. Observe for any change in your brain. Being giddy or a bit dizzy is natural at the beginning. Some people experience joy and laugh uncontrollably. If you are feeling giddy, it is a positive reaction, indicating increased blood supply and oxygen to the brain and opening the constricted blood vessels in your brain.

This easy-to-practice breathing technique deactivates Adrenaline, keeping your protective heart hormones circulating longer and providing multidimensional health protection.

The orbital flow of breath is an advanced technique and one of the most efficient breathing techniques you can practice anytime and anywhere. When used correctly, this technique can significantly enhance your vitality. When mastered, it is a powerful tool that can help you efficiently and quickly counteract stress.

The energy flow starts from your solar plexus in your lower abdomen. Then, it raises from the crotch alongside your spine to the back region of your head, climbs over the highest point of your skull, and descends to your upper lip. This is all part of the inhalation process. When you reach the peak of your whole breath intake, hold it for a second and then release your breath, exhaling and directing the energy from the bottom lip to the lower abdomen and your crotch. The exhalation usually lasts longer, about seven to eight seconds. This extended exhalation is not just a part of the breathing technique but also plays a decisive role in detoxifying your body at the highest possible rate. You move your body's energy alongside your own orbit and accelerate the movements of cerebrospinal fluid CSF, which nourishes and refreshes your brain.

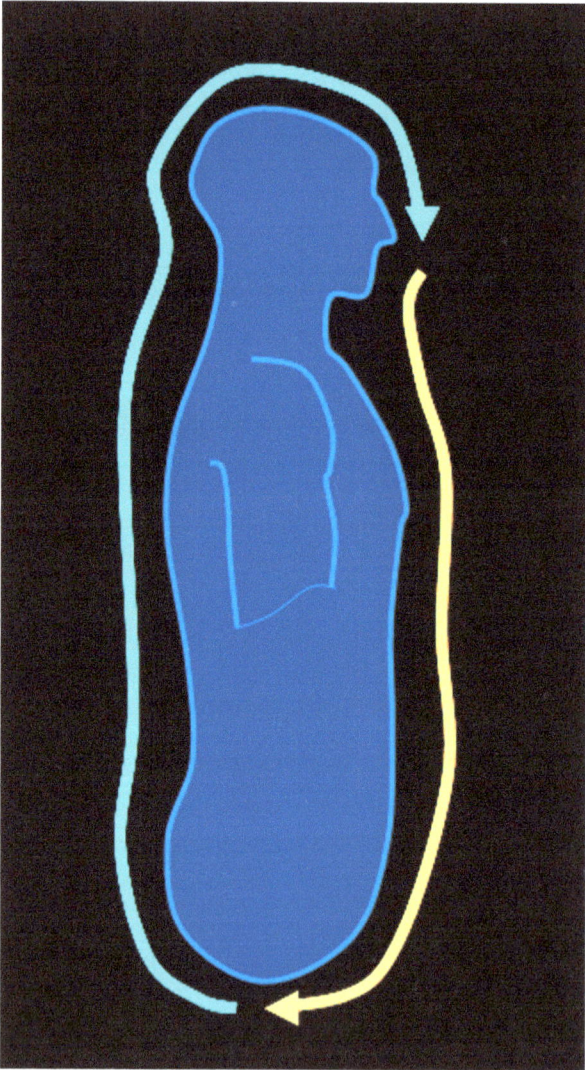

Picture 16. Microcosmic orbit by Bostjan46. Wikipedia.

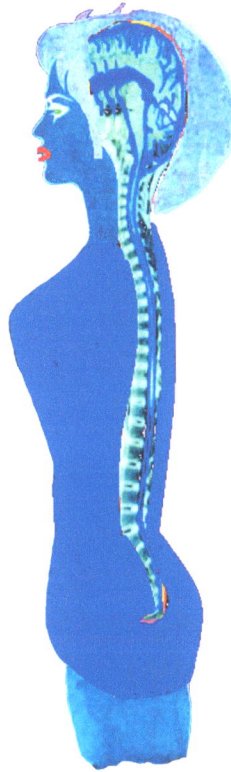

Picture 17, Cerebro-spinal fluid CSF.

Following the cerebrospinal fluid's gentle, rhythmic flow, similar to a dolphin's graceful movements, you can realize your body's endless pulsating state. Sometimes, you can be surprised by a wave of energy. It washes over your body from your head and shoulders to your toes. This bodily experience demonstrates the power of orbital breathing in energizing and revitalizing your entire body.

As you progress in your respiratory muscle training, you will feel the vitality streams in your energized body. This can eventually merge into an integrative quantum experience, a new quality in your body's feeling. Once you reach this experience, you will know you can achieve it again and again. This new perception of your body will be a joyful part of your orbital breathing, activating your brain and awakening your spine. Remember, where attention goes, the energy flows, and joy follows.

Several stress management techniques, such as meditation, yoga, journaling, or mindfulness are good for you. You can also connect with others in a support group or work with a professional counselor.

8

Cardiology for women

So God created human beings in his own image. In the image of God he created them. male and female he created them. Genesis Chapter 1, Verse 27.

Women face unique challenges and have specific needs when it comes to heart health. Their bodies, designed for beauty, comfort, and charitable, compassionate actions, are more sensitive to pain than men's due to internal reproductive female organs and feminine hormones.

Stress affecting your heart is a common factor in the modern life. It can have a profound impact on your feminine body, including also your brain, other internal organs and pelvic floor muscles. Your distressed heart will speak to you with the sign of palpitations and Angina pectoris. The referred pain can include your belly and the pelvis. The tension in the pelvic area can lead to pain and discomfort, including in the uterus, making it more challenging for women to manage stress and maintain integrity under stressful circumstances.

Stress and anxiety combined with pelvic pain can activate the pelvic stress reflex. It causes the pelvic floor muscles to contract, leading to increasing spastic pain and other bodily symptoms including your shallow breathing. Therefore, the manifestation of heart in distress in women can differ significantly from those in men.

The condition of a distressed heart is much more common in women than modern society has anticipated. It is vital for you to be aware of this fact, as it can guide you to proactive, inspired actions to detect early the risks for your heart in distress.

It may surprise you to learn that most of the heart and cardiovascular research, the major topics in Cardiology, including Angina pectoris and heart attack, has been performed on male populations. This has led to a potential lack of understanding of women's specific differences in heart and cardiovascular disease.

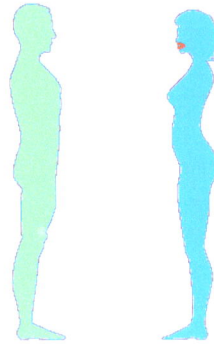

Picture 18. Woman and man.

More research is urgently needed on women's heart and cardiovascular health so that medical care experts, doctors, and affected women can better understand and address the unique challenges of feminine cardiology for the benefit of women. To make it very clear, all previous major studies on essential topics in cardiology, with the exception of the WARRIOR trial published in 2021, have been conducted with males, and the results have been unjustly transferred to the heart health of women.

The groundbreaking WARRIOR study, the first significant study in women's cardiology, revealed that aggressive therapy did not changed outcomes or provide benefits for women.

Experts on women's heart health and Cardiologists are actively dissecting the results of the WARRIOR study, a comprehensive investigation made with over 4000 women. They are particularly focused on vascular reactivity, inflammatory factors, and functional spasms as causes for the lack of positive outcomes from aggressive treatment in women.

It is truly exciting to see the WARRIOR study pave the way for a more comprehensive understanding of women's health in Cardiology.

However, there is hope that the scientific community, including cardiologists and researchers in women's health, will take a leading role in advancing our understanding of the feminine heart and women's heart health.

The Spanish Society of Cardiology, one of the first national cardiology organizations in the world, has published a document on cardiovascular disease in women just now, at the beginning of 2025. These groundbreaking guidelines, which summarize the views of a panel of experts organized by the Working Group on Women Health and Cardiovascular Disease, aim to raise awareness among healthcare professionals about preventing cardiovascular diseases in women. They highlight the differences between men and women, such as the unique risk factors and symptoms that women experience, and provide specific preventive recommendations tailored to the different stages of a woman's life.

Dr Antonia Sambola, coordinator of the writing on these guidelines in women's hearts and researcher at the Department of Cardiology, Vall d'Hebron University Hospital and Research Institute in Barcelona, Spain, told a Medscape Network platform that the early detection of heart health risk factors in women is critical.

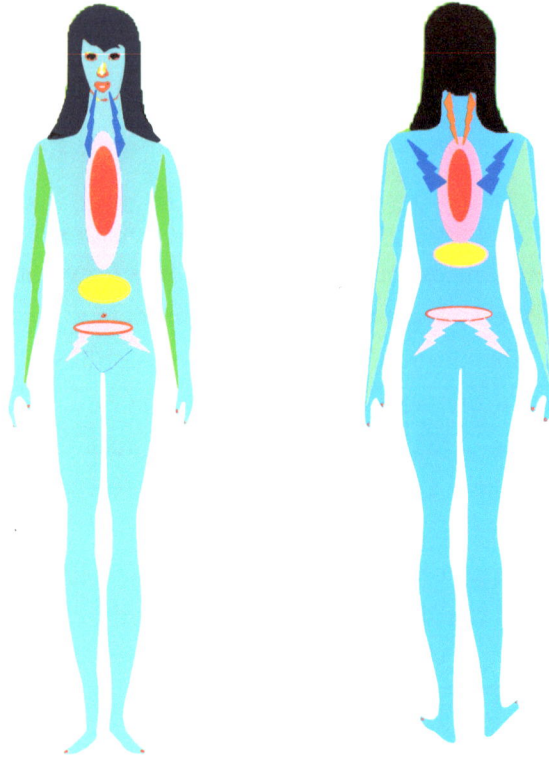

Picture 19. Localization of the referred heartache by women.

Women often experience different symptoms of heart distress. The presentation is not always dramatic, as portrayed in media, where a woman is shown clutching her chest. Instead, the symptoms can be subtle and more challenging to recognize. You may experience symptoms or discomfort in the stomach or abdomen rather than typical chest pain. It is not the classic presentation associated with a heart attack or Angina pectoris. Still, it occurs when your heart muscle does not receive enough oxygen-rich blood.

You need to be aware of these subtle symptoms and trust your instincts. As you know your body well, you may sense something is happening within your heart. Remember that common symptoms of heart distress in women include only insignificant chest discomfort , gentle heartburn, pelvic pain, and minor breathlessness.

It is important for you to know that Angina pectoris signs and symptoms can appear in your lower abdomen. You can feel pain, pressure, tightness, or discomfort in the pelvic region. The referred pain may radiate to your lower back, hips, or thighs. It worsens with exertion or stress, and significantly, this radiating pain improves with rest. Understanding these unique manifestations can better prepare you to recognize your troubled heart behind the veils hiding it.

Sometimes, mild breathing difficulties may be usual and not a cause for concern. A congested nose is one example. Another example is strenuous exercise, especially when you do not exercise often. If breathing difficulty is new or increases, it may be your heart. Furthermore, nausea, sweating, a feeling of impending to vomit, fatigue, and feeling giddy can be the first signs of a functional heart in distress.

While there are common risk factors that affect everyone, such as hypertension, smoking, high cholesterol, slow metabolism, and stress, you, as a woman, are destined to recognize your additional unique risk factors. Many women face challenges in conceiving a child due to a variety of factors, including environmental exposure to chemicals, pesticides, radiation, or heat, and the use of medications such as "The Pill" or those used to treat bacterial and sexually transmitted infections. It can affect their heart health negatively. High blood pressure, depression, and hormone imbalance due to polycystic ovary syndrome are further examples of cardiac risk factors. Pregnancy complications, early menopause, higher incidences of autoimmune diseases in women, and general body inflammation all of them can impact your heart health, too.

All these conditions cause not only cardiovascular stress but also significant amount of metabolic stress, and you are more susceptible to metabolic stress than any man.

Metabolic stress is an imbalance in your body caused by low oxygenation of the cells, nutrient deficiency, or excess. It is a serious issue that can cause low energy levels or even chronic fatigue. Metabolic stress leads to inflammation and tissue damage, highlighting the potential negative impact on your body and the profound weight of this condition.

Metabolic stress results from abnormal nutrient utilization and medication, as well as deficiency or excess of nutrients. More often, metabolic stress is a response to low energy levels that can occur when there is disequilibrium in your body's energy, leading to disruptions in the metabolic wheel.

Metabolic stress occurs when there is a need for more energy than it currently exists. It can be extreme emotional stress, or it can occur during exercise or a long-lasting intellectual effort. This results in an accumulation of waste products in your heart muscle and a build-up of toxins in your coronary vessels and heart, transforming a harmless narrowing into vulnerable and reactive plaque.

Toxic waste products of your distressed metabolism, like lactate and phosphate, enter the cerebrospinal fluid, brain, and spine and affect your muscles.

As a result, when you present yourself to a doctor, he is required to have special knowledge about Cardiology for women and cardiovascular and metabolic stress. Some professionals specialize in heart conditions, and very few in the unique needs you have as a woman with a distressed heart. Well, be a knowledgeable assistant to your Doctor regarding your heart being in distress.

Technically, suppose you, as a free woman, experience the threat of a heart attack. In this situation, you can feel fewer symptoms because your body size and your heart are smaller and equipped with thinner coronary blood vessels. You, as a busy woman, may also process certain medications differently because your liver is preoccupied with processing the female hormones. It takes away about 30 percent of your liver detox capacity. It is also the reason that women are stronger and longer exposed to alcohol intake than the man.

Other factors important for you and to keep it in your mind while visiting the health professionals:

- As a woman, you have an intelligent and delicate heart.
- Your nervous system influences your heart differently than a man's heart.
- Plaque formation in your coronary artery builds rather narrowing than a blockage.
- Your coronary vessels are more susceptible to a functional spasm.
- The pain receptors that alert women with heart in distress are differently functioning.

The signs of a threatening heart attack can be distinct for you as a woman, which can result in the fact that the development of a heart attack heart may go unnoticed until it is too late. It is essential for you as a woman to recognize that the most common symptoms of chest pain or discomfort, typically described as tightness, pressure, squeezing, or burning (Angina pectoris), can present themselves totally differently. Awareness of these differences can make you feel better informed and prepared to take action if necessary.

- If you feeling pain in the lower abdomen and pelvic area spreading to your hips and thighs due to activation of the pelvic stress reflex
- If you have a slightly burning sensation in the chest or upper abdomen
- If you are overwhelmed by cold sweats
- If you experience or discomfort in the chest or upper abdomen
- If you are feeling giddy or dizzy
- If you notice an irregular heartbeat or palpitations
- If you feeling nauseated
- If you experience weakness or pain or even discomfort in one or both arms, often described as pressure, ache, or stiffness that may come and go
- If you feel pain or pressure between your shoulders
- If you are surprised by mild shortness of breath
- If you constantly experiencing unusual intellectual fatigue
- If you feeling an unusual bodily weakness

it is the right time to seek medical support.

For women, a personalized approach to heart health is not just beneficial, it is imperative. This approach takes into account your unique feminine characteristics, family medical history, and current life situation to determine the most appropriate heart care. This tailored holistic care is designed to prioritize your well-being and achieve the best outcome for you.

Contemporary research confirms that women are at a greater risk of complications during invasive cardiac procedures such as balloon angioplasty, opening your narrowing, or blockage with a high-pressure plastic balloon. This underscores the critical need for female-specific approaches in cardiac invasive Cardiology. Women have been found to have more complications after undergoing balloon angioplasty, according to new research. Please remember what the WARRIOR trial revealed, there are no benefits of cardiological aggressive treatments for women.

The invasive procedure involves running a catheter through an artery to a heart blockage. But wait a moment. What happens if it is only a functional spasm and not a blockage? Still, a balloon is then inflated to open the artery and improve blood flow ? Often, a stent is also inserted to keep the artery open. But maybe the spasm could be released spontaneously by your body as a self-organizing system, or the specific medication could open it easily too.

The research found that complication rates were higher among women than men and even higher among younger women.

Overall, women were twice as likely to experience bleeding and vascular complications, and the younger women were also twice as likely to die in hospital. Complications more often occurring by women during cardiac interventions include heart attack, heart failure, stroke, and kidney. The research confirmed that females suffer more often specific complications after invasive procedures.

Leading cardiologists recognize the potential for significant improvement in heart care for women. They suggest that specific tailored strategies, such as personalized treatment plans, woman-specific risk assessments, and increased awareness of female-specific heart health needs, could lead to better outcomes for women.

9

Blood tests

The blood is God's sign bearing special significance. The blood signified a life had been given and sacrificed. Leviticus Chapter17, Verse 11.

Several blood tests can support the detection of your distressed heart.

The cardiovascular stress indicators.

According to the research, platelet count confirms that the platelets have remarkable adaptability concerning blood clotting. Platelet numbers can be counted through a complete blood examination test. These tiny cells, whose primary role is in clot formation and wound healing, exhibit a wide range of functions, from immunity to cell communication. When your coronary arteries are affected, platelets swiftly gather at the site to form a clot. Platelets attract a clotting substance called fibrin to form a net. The clot within a vulnerable plaque comprises platelets stacked in this net. This can make your existing narrowing critical and cause the symptoms of Angina pectoris.

A troponin test measures another protein released when the heart muscle does not receive enough oxygenated blood and could be damaged. Studies have shown that elevated troponin levels are also common after strenuous exercise in healthy women and in several other cardiac conditions.

Brain Natriuretic Peptide (BNP) is the hormone released by the heart in critical conditions, especially when the heart muscle is losing its strength. It helps the body to compensate for heart weakness. BNP is one of the powerful hormones produced by your intelligent heart. Heart weakness occurs when your heart becomes too weak or stiff due to multiple spasms in your coronary vessels. The reason for this can be the formation of the hibernating myocardium in the affected heart walls, preventing it temporarily from pumping normally. The most common causes for increased blood BNP are plaques due to coronary artery disease and not controlled high blood pressure. A result in your blood greater than 100 in one milliliter is abnormal.

The metabolic stress indicators.

Metabolic stress is the imbalance in your body caused by low oxygenation or even oxygen deprivation to cells. It needs special attention. It can cause inflammation and tissue damage, highlighting the potential negative impact on your body.

Metabolic stress can also result from abnormal nutrient utilization and medication metabolism. It can be caused by deficiency or excess nutrients. More often, metabolic stress is a response to low energy levels that can occur when there is disequilibrium in your body's energy, leading to disruptions in the metabolic wheel.

Metabolic stress happens when there is a need for more energy than it currently exists. It can be extreme emotional stress, strenuous exercises such as high-intensity interval training or marathon running, or a long-lasting intellectual effort like studying for exams or working on a complex project. This leads to a buildup of metabolites like lactate, phosphate, and hydrogen ions in the cerebrospinal fluid, brain and spine, heart muscle, and muscle cells.

Homocysteine, an indicator of metabolic stress, plays a significant role in heart health. It can be measured in your blood. Homocysteine is an amino acid that your body can not completely utilized in the presence of distress. Its high level indicates metabolic stress, and possible B12 vitamin, and Folate deficiency.

When your heart is distressed and you have a high level of Homocysteine, it contributes to blood clots and the increased risk of developing vulnerable plaques. However, the discovery of high Homocysteine can lead to positive changes. By supplementing Folate and consuming Vitamin B12-rich food or even starting the treatment of your metabolic stress with a B12 intramuscular injection, you can significantly improve your heart health and reduce your cardiovascular risks.

The inflammatory indicators of your heart in distress.

The most straightforward test is the C-reactive protein CRP in your blood. CRP is a protein produced by the liver. This remarkable organ plays a leading role in the body's inflammatory response. The level of CRP rises parallel to the level of inflammation in your body. A high-sensitivity C-reactive protein hs-CRP test, which is more sensitive than a standard C-reactive protein test, can detect smaller amounts of C-reactive protein in your blood. This sensitivity difference makes the hs-CRP test more effective in assessing the risk of developing vulnerable plaques.

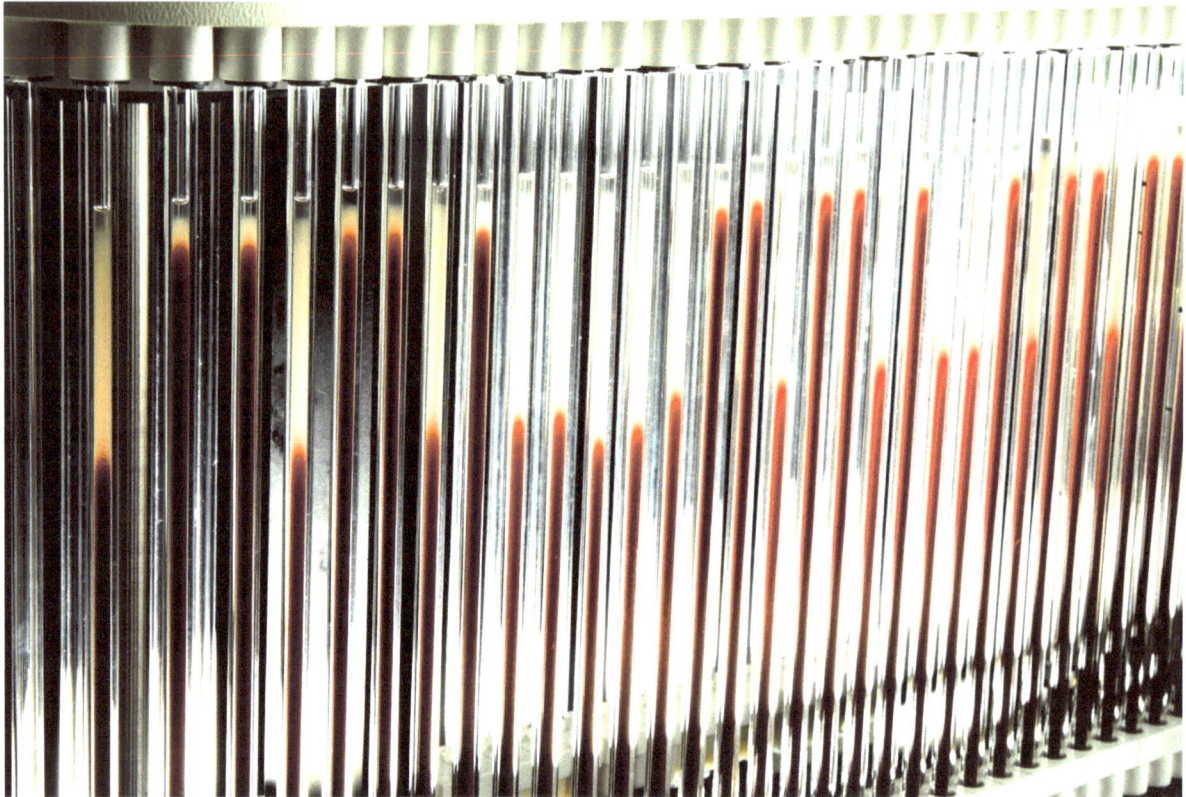

Picture 20. Westergren pipettes in automated StaRRsed ESR analyzer.
By MechESR. Own work.

The erythrocyte sedimentation rate (ESR) is a laboratory test that measures the speed at which your red blood cells settle to the bottom of a test tube. This test is a key indicator of your body's inflammatory response. A blood sample is placed in a chemical tube to prevent blood clots. The tube is left to stand upright, allowing the red blood cells to gradually fall to the bottom while the clear liquid plasma remains at the top. The ESR measures the rate at which the solid red and white cells separate from the liquid plasma and fall to the bottom of the test tube in millimeters per hour. If specific inflammatory proteins cover the red cells, they may stick to each other, causing them to fall more quickly. Therefore, a high ESR indicates the presence of inflammation in your body, making this test a vital tool in diagnosing heart health conditions.

Leukocytes, or white blood cells, are your immune system's first line of defense. Originating from your bone marrow, they tirelessly defend your body against infections and disease. This robust defense system should reassure you about your immune system's capabilities. When your immune system is under attack, such as during an infection, the number of white blood cells in your blood increases, a clear sign that your body is fighting back.

10

Cardiac imaging

*A*s long as the power in the eye enables you to behold the stars, as long you enjoy God's sunshine and breathe His air, so long will you yearn for knowledge. Paramahansa Yogananda.

Cardiac imaging refers to a range of techniques used to visualize your heart and its surrounding structures, including chest X-ray, ECG-electrocardiogram, echocardiography (ultrasound of your heart), cardiac computed tomography (CT scan), cardiac magnetic resonance imaging (MRI), nuclear medicine imaging (SPECT and PET), and CT coronary angiography. These techniques allow you and your doctors to get insight into the situation of your distressed heart, like valve problems, coronary artery narrowing, and heart muscle weakness.

There is an exceptional condition of the heart, also known as stress cardiomyopathy or heart in extreme distress. It produces similar symptoms and signs to a heart attack. Therefore, it is essential to rule out a heart attack first.

This process is not just about the doctor's actions but also about your active participation and understanding. Your inclusion in the decisions about the path of your diagnostics, which is necessary, is key to making you feel empowered and integral to your own healthcare. Your understanding and involvement in the chosen cardiac imaging procedure will help you feel confident about the process.

Your heart in distress is often associated with extreme emotional stressors triggered by a message about your serious health issue, tragic loss, surgery, or a traumatic event. The symptoms, which include chest pain, shortness of breath, palpitations, and feeling faint or sick, can be alarming. A combination of cardiac imaging tests has to be done to confirm the presence of your heart in distress, also known as stress cardiomyopathy.

1. Chest X-ray.

A chest X-ray is an imaging test that uses X-rays to create a picture of the organs and structures of your chest, including the heart and lungs. It is one of the most common cardiac imaging tests performed. A chest X-ray can show the size, shape, and location of your heart, lungs, airways, and blood vessels. It can help to discover conditions that affect your chest, heart, or lungs; however, it is important to note that it is not the most advanced test available in the 21st century, and there are other more comprehensive imaging techniques.

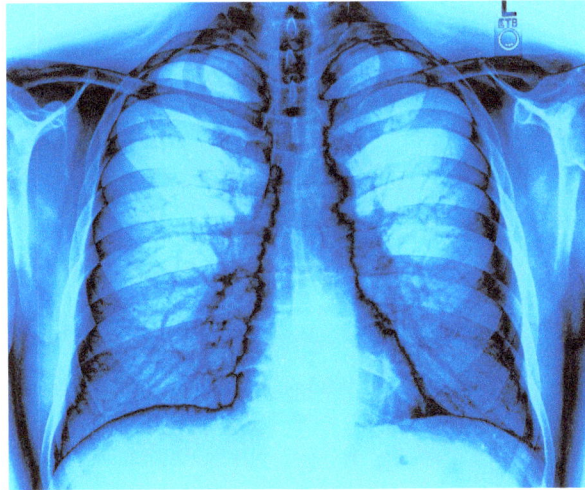

Picture 21. Chest X-ray PA inverted and enhanced.

By Stillwaterising, Wikimedia.

2. Electrocardiogram (ECG).

ECG is a powerful tool in the medical arsenal. Measuring the heart's electrical activity can swiftly confirm a distressed heart and, importantly, rule out the threat of an unfolding heart attack. The EKG shows abnormalities in its waves and a distinct normal pattern or an altered one showing a coronary artery spasm or blockage. It provides you and your Doctor a clearer picture of the situation in your coronary arteries.

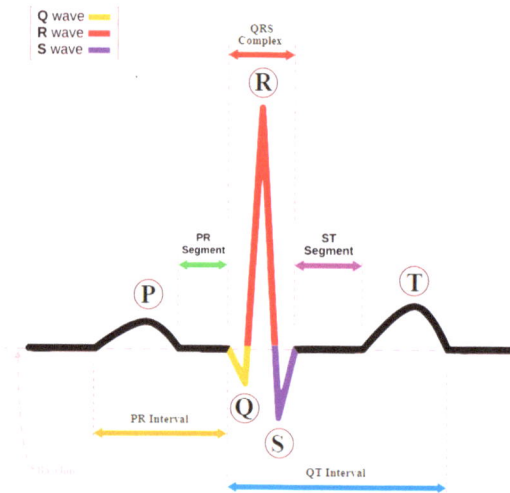

Picture 22. Created by Agateller (Anthony Atkielski).

Wikipedia

3. Echocardiography, or ultrasound of your heart (Echo).

It is a non-invasive and safe procedure. It uses ultrasound waves to create images of your heart, allowing doctors to visualize your heart while it's beating and assess your cardiac functions without any intervention. A small probe is placed on your chest to transmit and receive the heart-bounced sound waves. Unlike invasive procedures, an echocardiogram does not involve inserting instruments into the body or injecting a dye. It is a completely painless test that can help to discover a distressed heart or even stress cardiomyopathy. It shows how your heart is pumping blood and whether your heart muscle is weak or strained, all without causing any discomfort. An echocardiogram is the primary imaging test that allows doctors to visualize the characteristic pattern of heart muscle movement, particularly the less working parts of the heart muscle. It can also detect if your heart is over sized or displays a leaking heart valve.

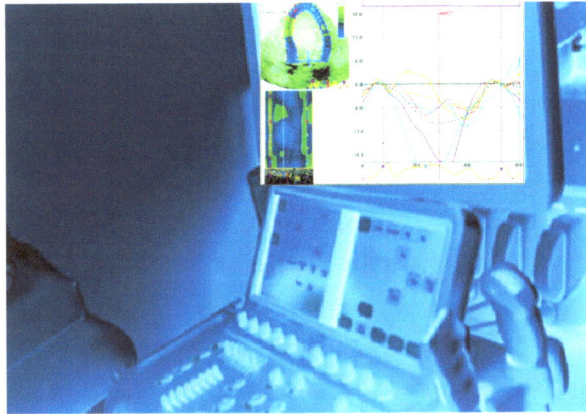

Picture 23. Echocardiogram.

Ultrasound of the heart is easy to perform. It can straightforwardly identify any abnormal movements in the heart chambers and recognize the characteristic 'ballooning' pattern seen in stress cardiomyopathy. Early recognition of your heart in distress through echocardiography will definitely determine better outcomes for you and help to predict which further heart imaging should be performed.

4. Coronary angiogram.

It can visualize your heart's blood supply. This makes it a helpful tool in confirming a heart in distress or even the stress cardiomyopathy, if with the ultrasound of the heart, MRI of the heart, or CT coronary angiography it could not be done.

During a coronary angiogram, a catheter is inserted into your artery in the groin or arm and guided into the heart. A dye is injected into the arteries, which makes them visible on X-ray images.

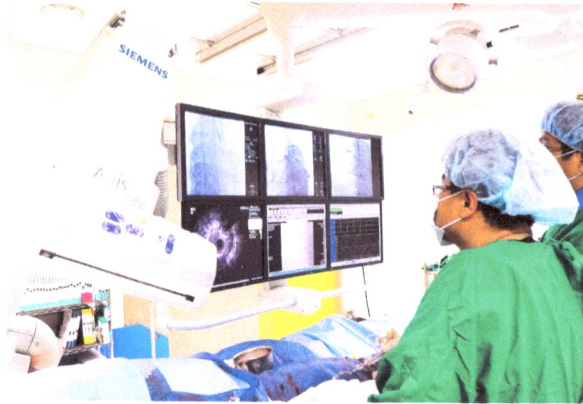

Picture 24. Angiography Room, Changwon Fatima Hospital, South Korea. By Jilly713 - Own work.

A coronary angiogram is an invasive procedure that uses X-rays to examine the heart's arteries, chambers, and coronary blood vessels. It's also known as a cardiac catheterization. It shows whether the coronary arteries are blocked or narrowed. The catheter is then moved into the left heart chamber, where a dye is injected. The dye makes the heart chamber visible on an X-ray, allowing the doctor to see if your heart muscle works properly. It is known as a ventriculography.

There are several concerning risks related to these procedures:

• Bruising or swelling at the puncture site.
• Allergic reaction to the dye or medications.
• Heart attack or stroke.
• Bleeding.
• Infection.
• Abnormal heart rhythms.

- There is a small risk of death by this procedure.

5. Nuclear ventriculography.

The nuclear technique, a safe and semi-invasive procedure, uses a radioactive tracer that is injected into your vein and remains in your body for a few days. This tracer attaches to red blood cells and travels through the heart. A specialized camera captures images of the red blood cells, which are then processed to reveal the heart's movement and the wall mobility of the heart chambers.

6. CT coronary angiography (CTCA).

There is also a semi-invasive procedure to visualize your coronary arteries. This is called CT coronary angiography.

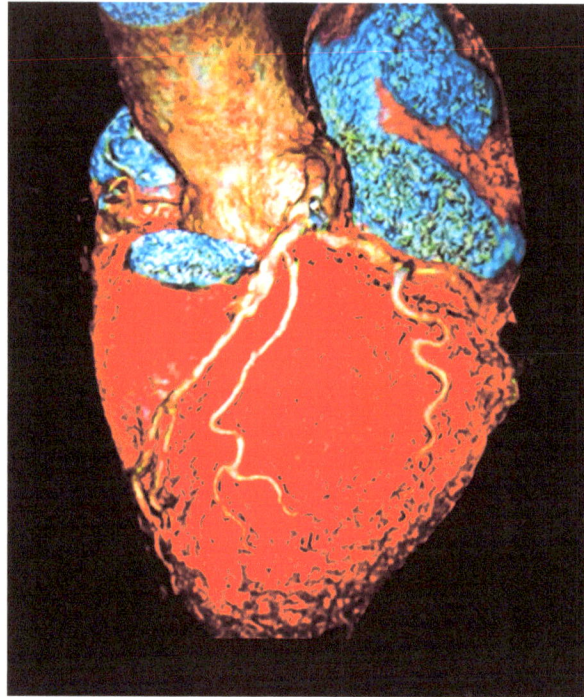

Picture 25. CT coronary angiogram CTCA.

A CT coronary angiogram (CTCA) is a semi-invasive procedure, known for its safety. During this process, a safe dye is injected into a vein in your arm or hand, and X-rays are used to produce images of your heart and coronary arteries.

CTCA is a powerful tool in diagnosing heart conditions, such as coronary artery disease, and plays a role in determining the most effective treatment options. It helps make other findings more likely or irrelevant by showing normal coronary arteries despite your cardiac symptoms. The injection of dye and using X-rays to take pictures of your heart make it a semi-invasive technique. Therefore, because your safety is the highest priority, you have to consider other, safer, noninvasive imaging techniques. One of them is the fully harmless magnetic resonance imaging (MRI).

7. **Magnetic resonance imaging (MRI).**

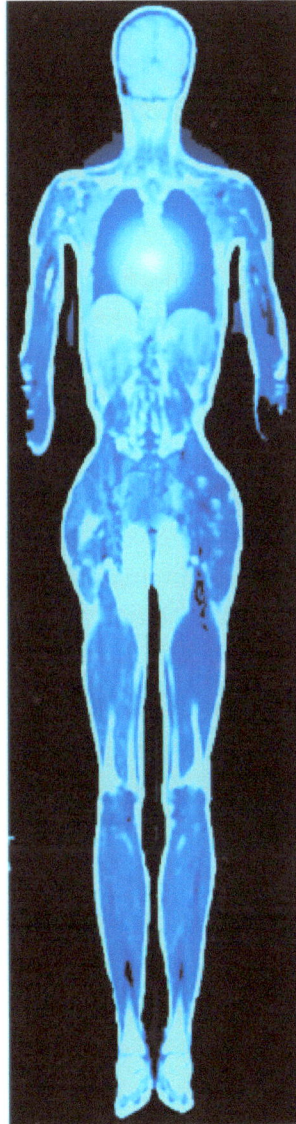

Picture 26. MRI of the full
feminine body.

Cardiac MRI, the safest imaging technique for your distressed heart, utilizes an external magnetic field to produce clear heart pictures. This safety reassures you, instilling confidence in the procedure. It enables precise visualization of your heart chambers, their shape, and possible enlargement.

Cardiac MRI, a non-invasive medical imaging technique, employs a magnetic field to generate highly detailed images of your heart and its surrounding structures. These detailed images provide valuable insights into the heart's size, shape, function, and overall health, delivering you and your Doctors precious knowledge about your heart condition.

But wait a moment. How can the human body be visualized using an external electromagnetic field?

An MRI scanner interacts with small, naturally occurring mini-magnets in your body's water. These mini-magnets are positively charged hydrogen atoms at the atomic level. Hydrogen, the universe's simplest and most abundant element, is pivotal in this process.

Consider this: a mere 1 milliliter of water contains an astonishing number of over 6 quintillion protons, represented by the number 6,000,000,000,000,000,000,000. This staggering number underscores the scale of an MRI scanner, visualizing the human body at the atomic level.

This multitude of mini magnets within your body all have random, chaotic orientations of their poles. MRI corrects them in one direction, creating a uniform alignment of the hydrogen protons. This process creates order within your body, which the MRI scanner can then capture in the form of detailed images. Seeing this order reflected in the excellent images of your body's internal structures is fascinating.

The strong external magnetic field penetrating your body and aligning the hydrogen protons in one direction is truly impressive. Your body responds positively to the order. Besides having excellent images of your heart chambers, MRI is an energizing bonus for your well-being. It is important to note that the MRI process is entirely safe, as the magnetic field is not harmful to the body when you are exposed to it for a short time.

Clinical presentation and physical exam are essential before any cardiac imaging. This includes medical history and physical examination. A detailed physical examination sometimes reveals low or high blood pressure, accelerated pulse rate, or other signs like a pale face, sweating, and tense muscles.

11

Development of the distressed heart

The LORD is near to the brokenhearted and saves those who are crushed in spirit. Psalm 34:18.

Historically, women have lived longer than men and have experienced fewer heart attacks due to protective hormones like estrogen and progesterone, as well as reduced exposure to stress. However, due to the challenging modern lifestyle, the heart has now become the source of the leading infirmity in women.

In the year 2023, about 4,000,000 women in the United States experienced heart attacks. Most of the affected women had no typical symptoms before the heart attack About 200,000 of these women suffered from heart in extreme distress known also as the stress cardiomyopathy. Many lives could have been saved if women had known their unique Angina pectoris symptoms.

Now you able to recognize early warning signs of your heart in distress. The healthcare professionals are in a position to identify underlying causes swiftly and timely to treat you knowing that coronary artery spasms or inflamed, vulnerable plaques are in the play.

The vital importance of Cardiology for women and the need for Doctors to be sensitive to women's heart health is evident within the medical system.

You can experience often untypical symptoms before a heart attack, and your heart attack may go unrecognized if you are sensitive enough to the women's Cardiology.

- If you experience fluttering feelings in the chest or palpitations, it is time to seek medical attention promptly.
- You can be surprised by a shortness of breath.
- Your sudden shortness of breath, general tiredness, or swelling of the feet, ankles, legs, or abdomen could indicate a heart health issue.
- You can feel pain, pressure, tightness, or discomfort in the lower abdomen. This referred pain may radiate to the back, hips, or thighs; it worsens with exertion or stress, and significantly, this radiating pain improves with rest.
- You can experience also pressure in the lower chest or upper abdomen.
- You can be surprised by sudden pain in your jaw or neck.
- You can feel nauseated or have a feeling to throw out.
- You could have dizziness or a feeling of fainting.
- The feeling of cold sweat can be a sign of your distressed heart language calling for your attention.
- You could have signs and symptoms of indigestion from your gastrointestinal tract, a cover up for the heart in distress.

If you experience these symptoms, it is your responsibility to seek medical attention immediately. Do not ignore them or try to tough it out. Your heart is too sensitive and too important to you to put it at unnecessary risk. By calling your doctor or going to the emergency room you are taking a proactive step towards your heart health.

Your decision to act in all these situations is correct.

Palpitations are not just a fleeting sensation; they can indicate potential heart issues. If you experience your heart fluttering or skipping beats, it is important to recognize these symptoms as they could be a warning sign and a threat to your heart health. In some cases, they may even indicate a potential heart attack. Sudden and excessive stress is a risk factor for your heart, leading sometimes to a condition known as a stress cardiomyopathy.

Adrenaline, a stress hormone, plays a significant role in the cascade of internal events in your body. It increases blood pressure and constricts blood vessels, demonstrating how stress can have immediate and significant effects on your heart, causing threatening signs and symptoms. An overproduction of Adrenaline can cause multiple spasms in your coronary arteries and, as a result, a rapid weakening of your heart muscle.

Stress is a profound challenge many women face, manifesting in dramatic ways. Yet, realize you have enough resilience and strength to encounter these challenges. Be a neutral quantum observer. Remember, no matter what happens, you can stay calm. Make the right decision based on your feminine intuition. You have only 10 seconds to decide if you will use your new knowledge and be like a solid rock or to react emotionally according to the generational "junk DNA" to be overwhelmed by the stressful impact on you.

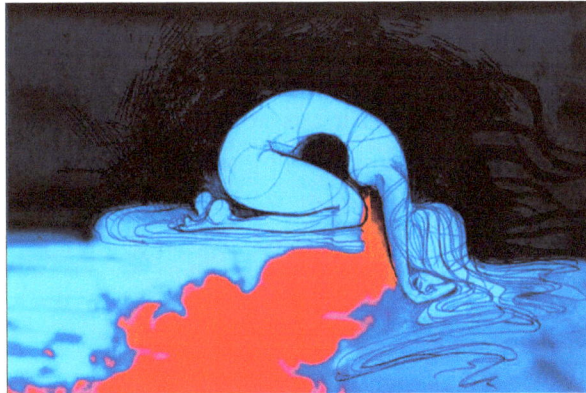

Picture 27. Artistic depiction of chronic fatigue symptoms (CFS) by a woman who has the condition, showing a woman slumped over with exhaustion. By Jem Yoshioka from Wellington, New Zealand. Wiki.

Emotional Symptoms: Stress can significantly affect your well-feeling, leading to anxiety, depression, anger, irritability, mood swings, and a sense of losing control. These emotional challenges underscore the need to identify your bodily signs of stress early. By doing so, you can adopt effective coping strategies, possibly regain control, and improve your emotional well-being. It can be also an impulse enhancing your life experience for a better future.

Intellectual Symptoms: Stress can manifest as forgetfulness, intense worry, difficulty focusing, and negative thinking. It is important to recognize these as manifestations of stress, not reflections of your true self. This understanding helps you to seek the proper support and manage stress effectively. It can also help you regain your clarity and stay focused.

Social Effects: Stress may lead to diminished relationship intimacy, feelings of isolation, family tensions, and an overwhelming sense of loneliness. These social aspects can intensify emotional distress. However, think about it and acknowledge that you are not alone in this world. Your helpers are already eagerly waiting to support you in your inner circle. Leveraging social support can be valuable in managing stress. It can provide you with a good feeling and reassurance. Realize that you have the connections you need when it matters most.

Hormonal Effects: Long-lasting distress can result in hormone imbalances, irregular periods, infertility, and even premature menopause. Additionally, it can compromise your immune system and heighten the risk of your heart being in distress. Hormonal imbalance is the root of higher levels of "bad cholesterol" and lower levels of "good cholesterol". It causes coronary blood vessel reactive changes, high blood pressure, and increased risk of blood clots, and most importantly, it accelerates plaque buildup in the arteries of your heart.

Endorphins, your body's natural painkillers, are released when your body feels stressed. Your body releases endorphins to help you survive. When you feel pain, nerves in your body send pain signals to your brain. Your brain releases endorphins to block the nerve cells receiving pain signals. This essentially turns off your pain, and therefore, you may experience a "silent" heart attack, where you do not have classical chest pain or any feminine forms of Angina pectoris but may have only unexpected fatigue.

Unique Stressors for Women: Women face distinct and specific stressors. Domestic violence, workplace inequality, and demanding family responsibilities are the challenges that intensify stress and impact your heart health. By knowing and addressing these unique stressors for women, you are not just taking proactive steps. You are becoming more aware and conscious of how you feel as a woman. It contributes to safeguarding your heart health and integrity. Remember that you, as the knowledgeable "quantum Observer," are changing reality, even without any other interaction.

When the harmless coronary artery plaque or narrowing becomes a vulnerable plaque, it becomes reactive and spasming. A vulnerable plaque is a type of plaque that is more risky and can lead to a heart attack or stroke. The spasms of major arteries supplying your heart muscle cause the bigger area of the heart to enter hibernation. This state of sleepiness is for your protection. Otherwise, your heart cells will die. In the hibernation, they are weaker but still alive. Your heart muscle cells are waiting for fresh blood and oxygen to restore their good functionality.

Another important aspect is the role of female hormones, particularly progesterone and estrogen, in heart health. These hormones play a big role in regulating the body's inflammatory response and keeping the coronary arteries open and wide.

Altered levels of these hormones, such as during menopause or pregnancy, can trigger a prolonged inflammatory response in your body and are significant factors contributing to dramatic signs and symptoms and the development of your distressed heart. A 'distressed heart' refers to a heart that is under significant and extreme stress, which can lead to a heart attack if not addressed.

12

A distressed woman's heart

It is not your passing thoughts or brilliant ideas so much as your plain everyday habits that control your life. Be directed by prudence, or wise forethought; be circumspect in all your actions; be careful, discreet, and sensible. Intelligence is a mark of God. Paramahansa Yogananda.

A heart in distress, a serious condition that primarily affects women, can lead to rapid weakening of the heart muscle. However, you need to remember that this condition is reversible. With appropriate medical care and a good supply of oxygen, your heart can heal and regain its normal function, offering hope for you. Your speedy recovery can be a good example of healing for those affected to follow your inspired actions.

The female heart, a complex and sensitive organ, is characterized by its smaller mass and size and unique functional, structural, genetic, and hormonal vulnerabilities. Understanding these feminine aspects of your heart can help you feel acknowledged as a woman and appreciate the complexity of your holistic heart health. You need to identify the potential triggers for the distressed heart early.

Your distressed heart can overwhelm you suddenly, often during unexpected and extremely stressful events. Uncontrolled negative emotions or receiving concerning news from a doctor about a serious illness or the need for surgery can be a triggering impulse. Commonly, financial losses, broken relationships, extreme violence, war experiences, post-traumatic stress disorder PTSD, sudden fear, the loss of close relatives, and significant climate events, such as earthquakes can put your heart in distress.

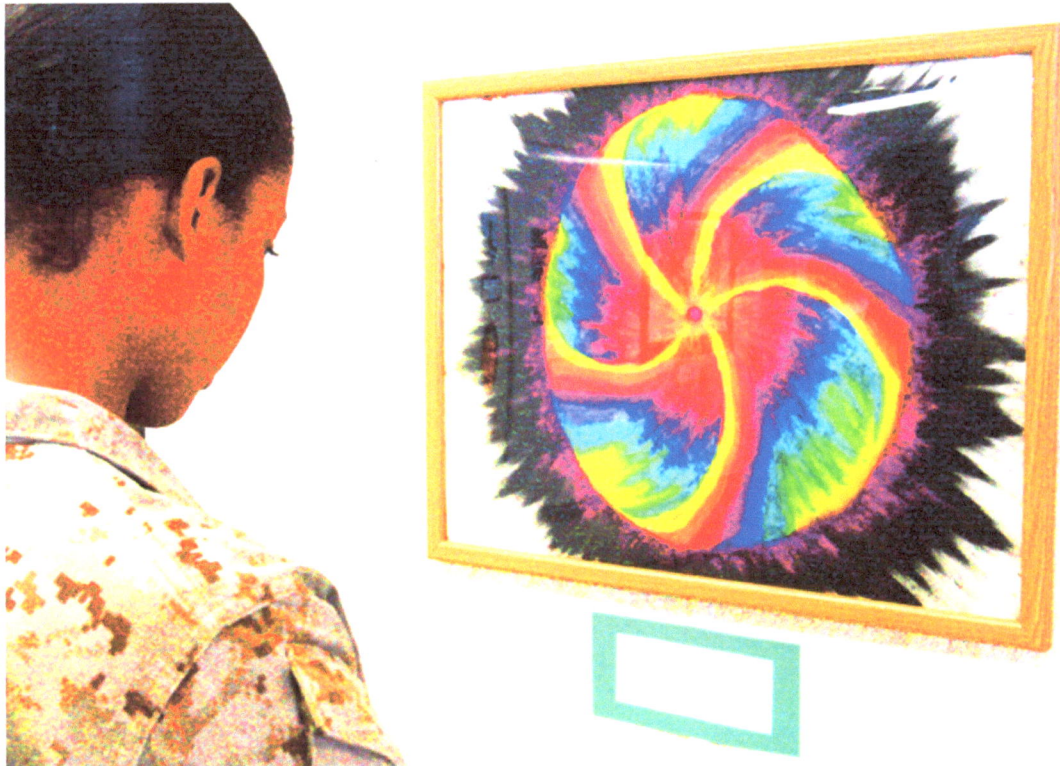

Picture 28. Service members use art to relieve PTSD symptoms. BY Cpl. Andrew Johnston - https://www.dvidshub.net/image/579803 Milford, Mass., native, Pfc. Jailene Delacruz, an embarkation specialist with Marine Light Attack Helicopter Squadron 167, 2nd Marine Aircraft Wing, reads a quotation from a Marine describing the painting on the wall and what it means to them. Paintings by Marines and sailors who attend art therapy to relieve post-traumatic stress disorder symptoms were displayed at an art expo May 3.

Even sudden positive surprises, like extreme happiness or receiving good news, can sometimes lead to what is referred to as a 'happy broken heart.' The symptoms and signs of this "happy" form of distressed heart are similar to those of a heart attack. They may include chest pain, all manifestations of feminine Angina pectoris, including your abdomen and pelvis, severe shortness of breath, unprovoked sweating, and feeling giddy or dizzy. They can appear suddenly within minutes or hours of the stressful, thrilling, and happy event.

By being aware of these symptoms and understanding the importance of seeking medical help, you can take preventative steps to protect your perfect heart health. Remember, seeking help is not a sign of weakness but a courageous step towards your perfect heart health.

As a woman, you have a deep understanding of your body and heightened sensitivity, which can lead to experiencing different symptoms of heart distress. This unique manifestation and sensitivity are important and should be acknowledged in the context of your heart health.

The dramatic portrayals in the media, where a woman is shown clutching her chest, your symptoms of heart in distress can be subtle and more differentiated making them difficult to recognize. You may have an instinct that something is wrong with your heart since you are very well familiar with your body.

Given the atypical female presentation of your distressed heart, you must receive specialized care from healthcare professionals who understand women's heart conditions. These professionals, including cardiologists and emergency room doctors, are trained to recognize the unique characteristics of women's heart health and are equipped to provide you with the necessary care. Their expertise and support can reassure you and guide you through the treatment process within the healthcare system.

Your distressed heart needs medical attention and must be addressed urgently. Remember, the symptoms can be intense. However, you need to know that your heart in distress is functional. It is vital to realize that one or more of your coronary arteries are spasming, producing insufficient blood supply to your heart muscle.

Your spasming coronary arteries are only narrowed and not blocked. The intensity of your emotional or physical reaction and lack of oxygen have caused it. You stopped your breathing following the bad news, outbreak of violence, or highly harmful messages.

Almost everybody on this planet Earth has plaques. So, your coronary arteries typically contain small plaques that do not significantly reduce blood flow and oxygen supply to your heart muscle. However, when a coronary artery spasm occurs, it narrows and constricts your coronary vessel, leading to a reduction in blood supply to your heart. The spasm does not take place because your artery is clogged. It happens due to a functional change caused by a significant lack of oxygen, often in distressed situations. Your breathing became shallow and not sufficient.

It is important to note that nearly everyone, including children, has some plaques in their arteries at particular times in their lives. These plaques are buildups of fats, cholesterol, debris, fragments of bacteria and viruses, and other substances that accumulate in the walls of the heart's arteries, just a "stuff."

While this buildup can lead to slight narrowing, it does not necessarily decrease blood flow or oxygen supply. Having a plaque in your heart does not automatically mean you will experience symptoms of your feminine Angina pectoris or a heart attack. A plaque must become vulnerable, active, and spasming to cause any damage to the heart. Extreme stress and emotional overload can trigger this activation.

Understanding the nature of your heart in distress can help you recognize and respond effectively to the alarming signs. It also offers hope for a full recovery.

13

Treatment and healing

*L*ord my God, I called to You for help, and You healed me. Psalm 30:2:

Your heart in distress can be described as an instant negative heart remodeling. This urgent situation requires your attention. In this process, your heart undergoes structural and geometrical changes caused by extreme stress. In a nutshell, your healing is to restore your heart to its original healthy condition before an unexpected and overwhelming change has occurred.

As you take healthy steps towards healing, such as receiving medication, doing your orbital breathing regularly, eating a balanced diet, and managing stress, you are restoring day by day your heart's normal shape, softening its hardened structure, bringing back its natural size, and regaining its once-perfect metabolic flexibility.

Please remember that you are also participating in a natural healing of your body, and your inspired actions will lead to the full recovery of your heart. Understanding the language of your body is fundamental. Your new knowledge of Cardiology for women must result in decisive actions, giving you a positive shot of emotional energy and bringing you joy of accomplishment.

Rest assured that conventional medicine is a safe and highly effective tool in your fight against heart in distress. Its proven track record can instill a sense of security and confidence in your actions.

Knowing that your coronary vessel causing your condition is only functional narrowed, not blocked, can support your steady course in your healing journey and avoid unnecessary panic.

Nitroglycerin effectively helps your distressed heart because it can resolve the spasms in your heart's blood vessels in seconds or minutes. These spasms are often caused by the release of excess Adrenaline, a hormone that can constrict your coronary arteries. The re-opening of your arteries is an uplifting experience because you realize instantly that your healing is possible.

The plaques, a buildup of fats, cholesterol, debris, fragments of proteins, dead cells, and other 'stuff' such as calcium and cellular waste, in the artery walls can become inflamed, reactive, and spasming. Generally speaking, you, as a woman, are more susceptible to spasms of the coronary artery despite having fewer cardiac risk factors.

While healthcare professionals play a fundamental role in a successful healthcare system, your personal engagement and expanded knowledge are equally important. By becoming a "knowledgeable quantum observer"of your body and your healthcare environment, you can develop the confidence needed to take charge of your treatment plan for your heart in distress.
No one understands your heart's impressive ability to fight illness and maintain your perfect heart health better than you do. Traditionally, Western medicine has taught us that our bodies are mainly unchangeable and primarily fixed in form. Beside from noticeable changes like weight gain or loss and variations in strength and flexibility, it has been widely accepted that your organs only change due to age-related deterioration. However, recent scientific discoveries about heart regeneration and brain plasticity reveal that you can recover from trauma pretty quickly if you allow your body to adapt its functionality according to the actual demands.

Remarkably, your heart has an incredible capacity to adapt, transform, and renew itself, far surpassing even the brain's plasticity. As a liberated woman who understands her body as a self-organizing system, you have a mission to unlock your heart's intelligence, which embodies its innate wisdom and adaptability. Doing so will allow you to re-evaluate your heart's role in your body and prioritize your intelligent heart needs in your new lifestyle.

Pharmaceuticals

Pharmaceuticals are medicines and medical devices used to prevent, treat, or cure disease. They can also diagnose conditions or promote well-being. The pharmaceutical industry researches, discovers, develops, produces, and markets pharmaceuticals.
Pharmaceuticals are available by prescription from a registered healthcare professional or over-

the-counter from pharmacies and other retail outlets. When used appropriately, pharmaceuticals are an essential pillar of public health.

The pharmaceutical medicines used in treatment of your heart have some side effects, but remember that. you need to take them only for a short time to bridge the time of emergency with your distressed heart.

1. Nitroglycerin.

Nitroglycerin has a fascinating history, shaped mainly by the contributions of the engineer Alfred Nobel. He developed its use as a blasting explosive by mixing it with an absorbent, particularly 'Kieselgur,' a form of silica from the soil. He named this explosive dynamite and patented it in 1867. From his amassed fortune, he funded the Nobel Prize Foundation. Believe it or not, Mr Nobel suffered from a heart condition marked by intense chest pain (Angina pectoris), and his doctor prescribed him Nitroglycerin. It is a powerful medicine that opens the spasm of the coronary vessels by converting your body directly to NO. Nitric oxide was proclaimed the "Molecule of the Year" by the prestigious journal *Science* in 1992. Then, the research about NO was awarded the Nobel Prize in Medicine in 1998.

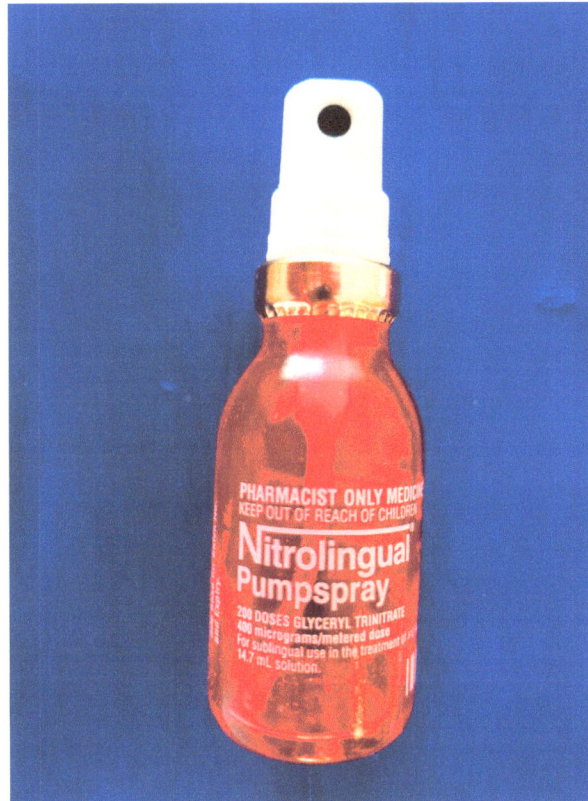

Picture 29. Nitroglycerine spray.

Who could have predicted 25 years ago that NO, a common pollutant from car exhaust fumes, would make such a medical career? It has remarkable benefits for your body. It resolves coronary spasms, protects your heart from getting weak, stimulates your brain, and even can kill bacteria. Despite its short 10-second life span, it is a universal positive agent, a fact that is often overlooked. It regulates the opening of your coronary blood vessels, determines your blood pressure, can prevent any kind of Angina pectoris, and stops the formation of blood clots.

It is useful to know that Nitroglycerin, the red heart spray, converts in your body directly to Nitric Oxide (NO). Nitrolingual spray is available in every pharmacy. NO is also vital for your brain function. It links to a good memory and is a key player in your body's defense system. NO aids in fighting infections because it is toxic to invading bacteria and parasites when produced by your immune cells. This incredible molecule is also utilized by blood cells to defend the body against tumors, making its role in your body genuinely indispensable.

Nitroglycerin can be used to treat symptoms of extremely distressed heart, also known as stress cardiomyopathy. It helps widen coronary blood vessels and improve blood supply to the heart. Nitroglycerin is a potent solution for stopping Angina pectoris pain. However, its effectiveness depends on the correct administration. Spraying it in the mouth or under the tongue can lower blood pressure, so it is important to monitor the BP and administer it correctly in a lying position.

Some patients have been applying Nitroglycerin as a patch on the skin before they used Nitrospray. It has inspired them to use the Nitroglycerin spray differently. Spraying their chests with Nitrospray has helped to disappear their Angina pectoris and relieved their heart palpitations, but it did not lower their blood pressure. They reported that this method provided more comfort and helped them avoid the sudden decrease in blood pressure when taking it in the mouth.

Nitroglycerin is not only effective in the prevention of Angina pectoris. It is not only an emergency medication. It can be a tool you can apply just before daily activities. This knowledge about Nitrospray can help you to take control and prevent episodes of discomfort in the heart region when your heart would like to fall in distress.

There is a widespread agreement among major international cardiac societies that Nitroglycerin is a first-line treatment for (Angina pectoris). They recommend its use for Angina pectoris episodes due to its ability to rapidly dilate coronary blood vessels and improve blood supply to the heart.

This global agreement about the use of Nitroglycerin includes the European Society of Cardiology, the American College of Cardiology, the American Heart Association, the American College of Physicians, the American Association for Thoracic Surgery, Preventive Cardiovascular Nurses Foundation of Australia & Cardiac Society of Australia and New Zealand, and the Asian Pacific Society of Cardiology, which represents 23 cardiology societies in the Asia-Pacific region. The Indian Heart Association and the Chinese Society for Cardiology also support this practice. This widespread support for Nitroglycerin can make you more confident and secure in its daily application.

2. Angiotensin-converting enzyme ACE.

ACE drugs counteract stress, treat high blood pressure (hypertension), and strengthen the heart by making its work easier. ACE inhibitors block the stress agent Angiotensin in the body. Less Angiotensin relaxes blood vessels and lowers blood pressure.

3. Beta-blockers.

Beta-blockers block the action of Adrenaline, slow the heart rate, and make the heart pump blood around the body more easily. They can also help promote heart recovery. Their effectiveness was demonstrated by their use by musicians, public speakers, actors, and professional dancers to manage performance anxiety and tremors during auditions and public performances. The performers obtained Beta blockers from friends and colleagues.

4. Blood-thinner medicines.

When extreme stress affects your heart, leading to stress cardiomyopathy, it is important to understand the potential risks. The heart walls may move less, slowing down blood flow and increasing the risk of clots. However, the use of blood thinners can provide reassurance, significantly reducing the risk of a blood clot breaking loose and causing a micro-stroke.

5. Oxygen therapy.

Oxygen therapy is a part of the treatment for your heart in distress. It increases oxygen in your blood, which in turn helps to release the spasms in your coronary artery system. Oxygen therapy increases oxygen in the blood and oxygenation of the internal organs, heart, lungs, brain, and liver. It is paramount in treating and preventing complications from your extremely distressed heart and can be applied in a hospital environment and at home using a home oxygen concentrator.

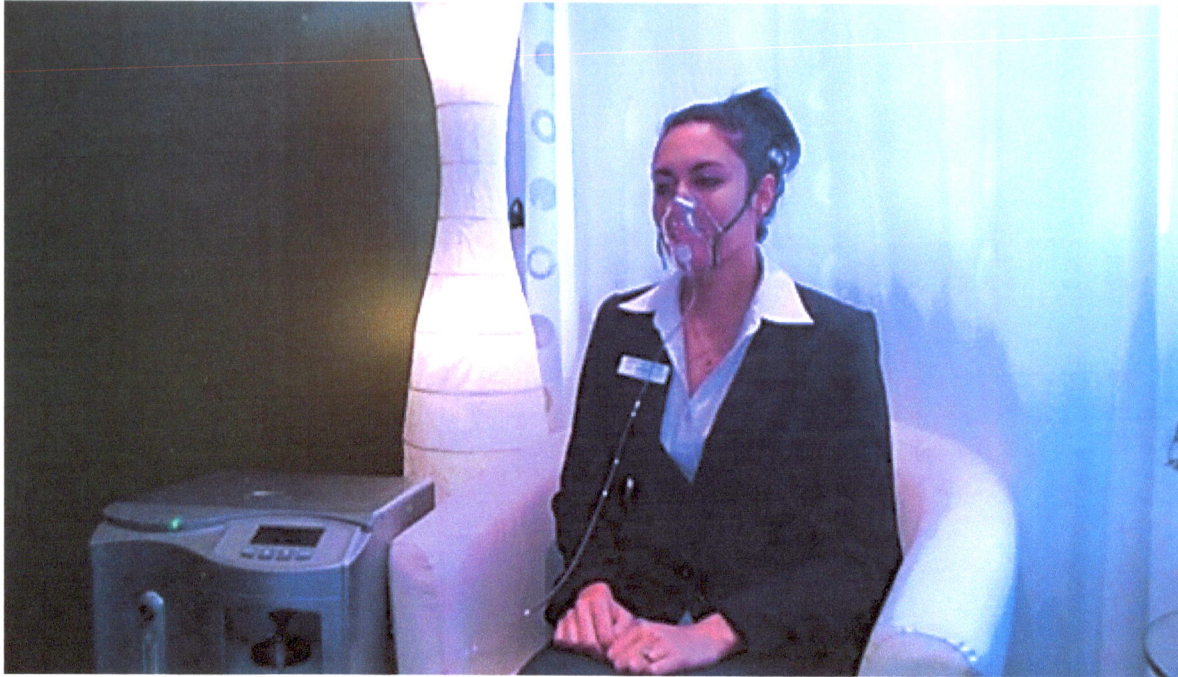

Picture 30. Oxygen therapy with oxygen concentrator.

Using the correct technique, such as abdominal diaphragmatic breathing, you can significantly increase the impact of the oxygen-enriched air you inhale via an oxygen mask, which will benefit your precious heart.

Portable oxygen concentrators represent a modern and safe approach to oxygen therapy. These devices directly separate oxygen and nitrogen using a molecular micro filter system called Zeolite or a special membrane and provide a convenient and reliable source of oxygen. They can deliver 5 to 10 liters of oxygen in a minute.

6. High-flow oxygen therapy.

High-flow oxygen therapy, also known as heated humidified high-flow oxygen therapy, is a breathing support treatment that delivers a mixture of oxygen and air through a nasal cannula at a flow rate of up to 60 liters per minute, is particularly beneficial for your distressed heart and resulting and heart weakness.

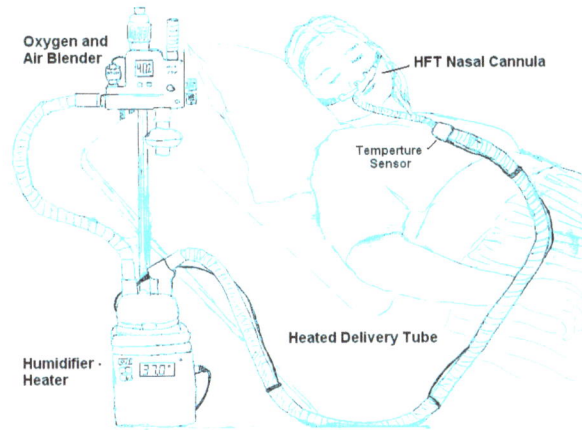

Picture 31. Strangecow at English Wikipedia - Artist: Strangecow. Offered for free use into the public domain.

Nutriceuticals

Nutriceuticals are food parts. They have been used as plant-related extracts or herbs with health benefits. They are a fusion of nutrition and pharmaceutical preparation. They are formulations of nutrients that lower "bad cholesterol" and aid in preventing, treating, and healing distressed hearts.

A compounding chemist can formulate and prepare them under the strict regulation of the Therapeutic Goods Act TGA in Australia.

The Food and Drug Administration (FDA) regulates nutriceuticals as dietary supplements in the United States. They are a broad category of products that includes vitamins, minerals, herbs, and amino acids.

Berberine.

Berberine is a natural compound that comes from the herb known as the Chinese gold thread. It lowers "bad cholesterol".

It also has multiple other effects, including anti-allergic, supportive of your heart rhythm, and cardioprotective. Some studies have shown its anti-tumor potential.

Red yeast rice.

Red yeast rice, a natural solution, can effectively lower cholesterol. It is derived from fermenting rice with a yeast known as Monascus purpureus. This dietary supplement contains monacolin K, which is similar in action to the Statin. It can also improve the function of blood vessels in the lining and increase the flexibility of coronary arteries. In the United States, red yeast rice is an alternative to Statin therapy to treat mild to moderate high cholesterol.

Policosanol.

Policosanol, a blend of higher primary aliphatic alcohols derived from sugar cane wax with octacosanol as its primary component, has been shown to lower cholesterol. This mixture effectively reduces cholesterol production in the liver. It enhances the breakdown of low-density lipoprotein LDL, which is coined as 'bad cholesterol". It also reduces the stickiness of blood cells, known as platelets. Notably, policosanol offers potential relief for leg pain during exercise due to poor blood flow.

Bergamot.

Bergamot, a citrus fruit, has been shown to lower cholesterol levels. Citrus bergamia, the Bergamot orange, is a fragrant citrus fruit the size of an orange, with a yellow or green color similar to a lime, depending on ripeness.

Genetic research into the ancestral origins of extant citrus cultivars found Bergamot orange to be a probable hybrid of lemon and bitter orange. Studies have indicated that Bergamot extract reduces "bad cholesterol" and increases "good cholesterol". Bergamot lowers cholesterol by inhibiting the intestines' cholesterol intake and reducing liver cholesterol production.

Oriental raisin tree.

Current research indicates that the Oriental raisin tree, also known as Hovenia dulcis extract, can significantly lower cholesterol levels. This is primarily due to its active compound, dihydromyricetin (DHM), effectively reducing your LDL, the "bad cholesterol."

In traditional medicine, the Oriental raisin tree has a rich history of use for various health concerns. One of its key benefits is its positive impact on liver health, which is closely linked to cholesterol management in your body. This connection underscores the comprehensive health benefits of this natural remedy for your well-being.

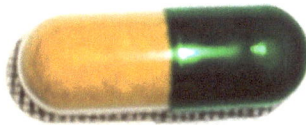

32. Nutriceutical mega-capsule.

Imagine these valuable nutriceuticals compounded into one, single capsule. This mega capsule can be formulated by any compounding chemist. Mega is not based on the capsule's size but because of its significant positive impact on the lipid profile and strong anti-inflammatory potential.

Acupuncture.

Acupuncture, a key treatment in traditional Chinese, Japanese, and Korean medicine, is a therapeutic procedure that is highly effective in regulating your bodily functions. By utilizing the energy channels and specific entry points to your body, acupuncture helps to maintain a balanced and healthy body. It is also known for calming the mind and body by stimulating the release of natural opioids known as Endorphins. Effectively, acupuncture reduces stress in your heart and brain.

14

Medical acupuncture

Create in me a pure heart, O God, and renew a steadfast spirit within me. Psalm 51, Verse 10.

The network of energy channels or meridians is the cornerstone of acupuncture in traditional medicine. You will be surprised to know that Chinese traditional medicine has roots in ancient China and a medical history that dates back more than 2000 years.

Dr. Hua Tuo, a renowned Chinese acupuncturist, significantly contributed to acupuncture, surgery, and anesthesia. He was born in the year 108 after Christ and reached the age of 100 because Dr. Hua Tuo's expertise went beyond acupuncture. He combined acupuncture with other traditional Chinese medical practices, such as moxibustion (burning of special preparation of Artemisia Mugworth on the acupuncture needles), Chinese herbal medicine, and medical exercises, demonstrating a profound and holistic understanding of the human body.

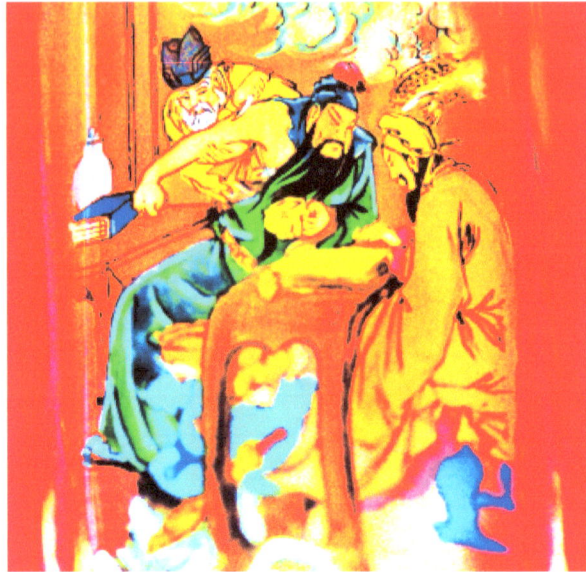

Picture 32. The famous Acupuncturist Dr Hua Tuo.

His legacy lives on through the 48 acupuncture points he discovered to be located along the spine, which are still used by practitioners today. These points are highly effective in treating conditions related to the spine and major internal organs, instilling confidence in the practice of acupuncture and reminding us of his enduring impact on the development of traditional Chinese medicine.

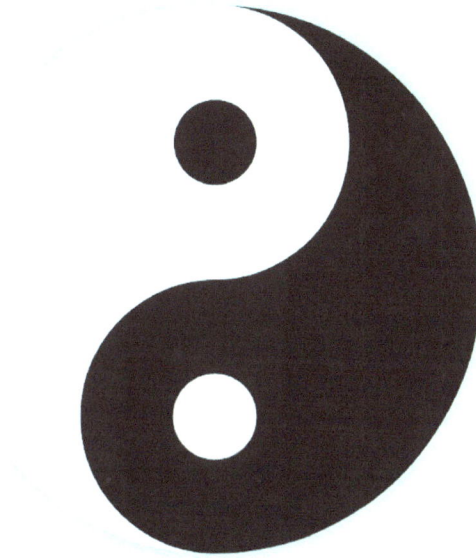

**Picture 33. Yin and Yang. By Klem, this vector image
was created with Inkscape by Klem, and then manually
edited by Mnmazur. Wikipedia.**

The Book of Change known as "I Ching" is significantly connected to traditional Chinese medicine because its principles, particularly the of Yin and Yang categories and the cyclical nature of the universe, provided the foundational framework for many aspects of the acupuncture and traditional medicine.

According to the knowledge and scientific studies of the 21st century, acupuncture is a quantum medical intervention. The target of acupuncture is the energy network, acknowledged as the living system of bio-information and energy that ensures the perfect functionality of your body. Understanding how these energy channels operate is a fascinating aspect of holistic medicine, enhancing the benefits you receive from acupuncture.

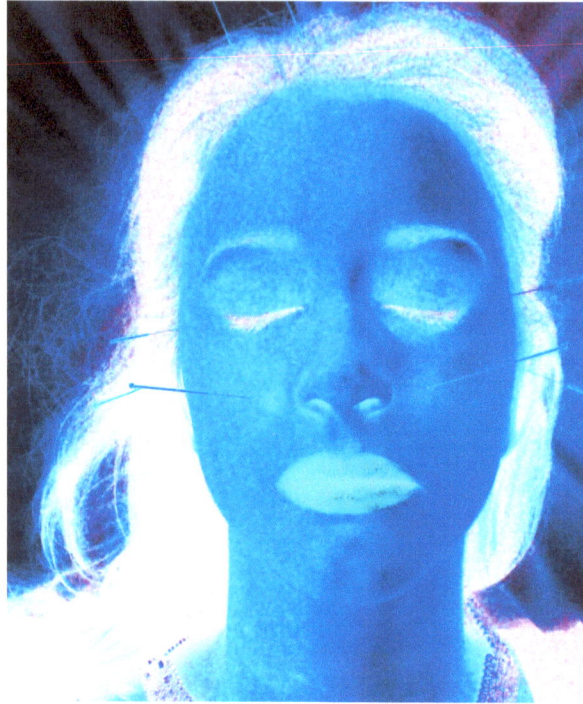

Picture 34. Medical acupuncture.

The energy channels are the framework for massage, reflexology, and acupuncture therapy. The therapists apply this knowledge in every holistic clinic and surgery.

While some Chinese medicine historians state that 'meridian' may not be the most accurate term for these energy channels, it has become the widely accepted translation.

The energy channels in your body are linked to major sensory and motor nerves, pathways for vital energy flow. According to 21st-century medical research, they are connected with your brain, heart, and spinal cord. The solar plexus in the belly and the pelvic plexus below your navel are specialized neuronal centers that team with your heart, brain, and spine through the energy channels. Is it not cool to understand your bodily energy systems more in detail?

It is truly fascinating, and you will be surprised to learn that your body communicates wirelessly through electromagnetic waves, much like your mobile phone. This exchange of vital information between your mind, brain, nerve cells, neurons, and internal organs, all of which have structures similar to antennas, is a process that, once understood, can inspire you. These structures are responsible for receiving, collecting, sending, and transmitting signals.

It is your mind that is in charge of this wireless communication process. It sends out commands that are received by the muscle cells' antennas. The nerves, acting locally, then translate these messages from your mind to your muscles and internal organs via electrical currents. Understanding this process is a key to better comprehending your bodily functions, from relaxing your muscles to accelerating your breathing.

Be inspired by the fact that your heart masters your bodily communication; its tools are your hands. What intention is in your heart will be performed by your hands.

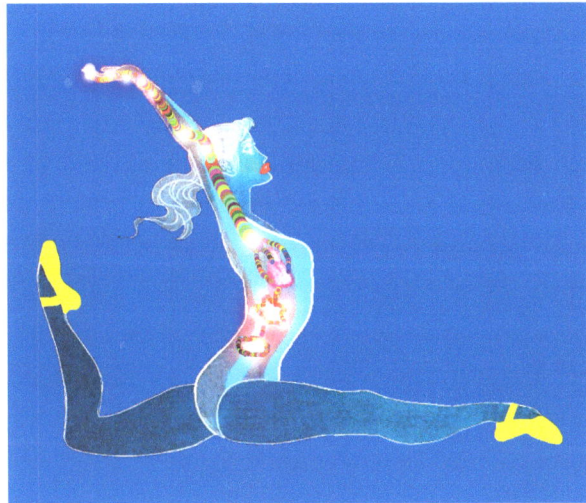

Picture 35. Heart energy channel. The solar and the pelvic plexus are displayed, and their links to the heart are visible.

The heart energy channel starts in your heart in the middle of your chest. It then travels down from the armpit and breaks through to the outside of your body, running down alongside your arm and forearm. It ends on the top of your small finger.

The heart energy channel within your chest provides internal branches down to your small intestine, solar plexus, and pelvic plexus. Another branch goes up to the eyes and tongue. The heart energy channel contains nine acupuncture entry points.

Your body houses two types of internal organs: the five primary internal organs, which serve as energy producers known as the yin organs, and their partner organs, which distribute the vital bio-energy created by the primary organs, known as the yang organs . Your heart partners with the small intestine, the lungs with the large intestine, the liver with the gall bladder, the kidneys with the urinary bladder, and the spleen with the stomach. This teaming of the internal organs means that your ten internal organs are connected to ten energy channels on each side of your body, forming a complex network.

Two additional energy channels are connected to your body's lymphatic system. The first is the energy channel of the pericardium, the sac surrounding the heart. The second is the triple energizer energy channel. This channel is connected to lymphatic structures and lymphatic vessels in three cavities of your body: chest, abdomen, and pelvis.

Traditional medicine takes a holistic approach, viewing your heart as the central organ of the human body. It governs your physical body and is fundamental for your spirituality.

The brain is not just another organ. In traditional Chinese medicine, it is regarded as a special organ. It connects to its own energy system, represented by two extraordinary energy channels: the conception energy vessel travels down in the front-line of your chest, tummy and pelvis of your body and the governing energy channel running alongside the spine and head on the back of your body. This unique role of the brain in connecting with each part your body's and building the microorbit of your breathing is a key aspect of traditional medicine.

In traditional Chinese medicine, the hollow, moving, or transporting organs are the yang organs. They receive, digest, transmit water and food, and eliminate waste. This contrasts with the yin organs, which produce, store, and transform vital substances. The yang and yin classification provides a clear understanding of the function of the internal organs in your body.

The ten energy channels are vital, influencing internal organs and enabling profound natural and functional changes. For instance, when balanced, the heart's energy channel can regulate blood circulation and influence emotional well-being. In contrast, the liver energy channel can improve your vitality and accelerate digestion and detox.

The governing and conception vessels merge at the mouth, lips, and tongue to form a brain energy channel, which guides the energy during orbital breathing. This technique enhances the flow of energy in the body and cerebrospinal fluid circulation in the spine canal and the brain.

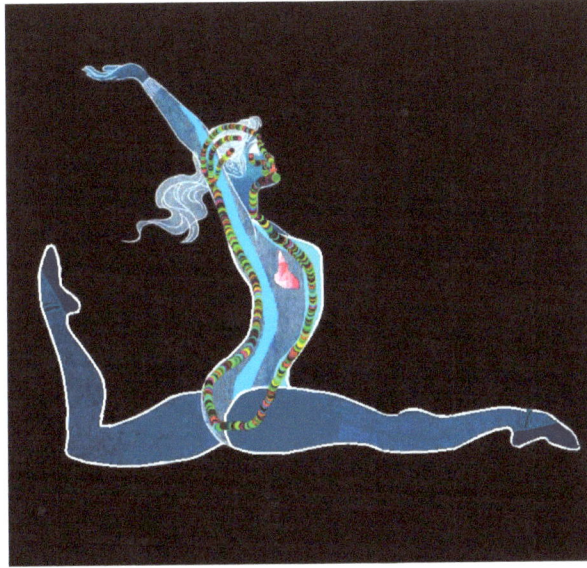

Picture 36. Brain energy channel.

Acupuncture is a key treatment in traditional European, Chinese, Japanese, and Korean medicine. It targets the body as a self-organizing system with its energy channels, which bridge internal organs and the body's connection to nature and its immediate environment. Acupuncture is a therapeutic procedure that utilizes the body's energy channels and their specific entry points to regulate bodily functions.

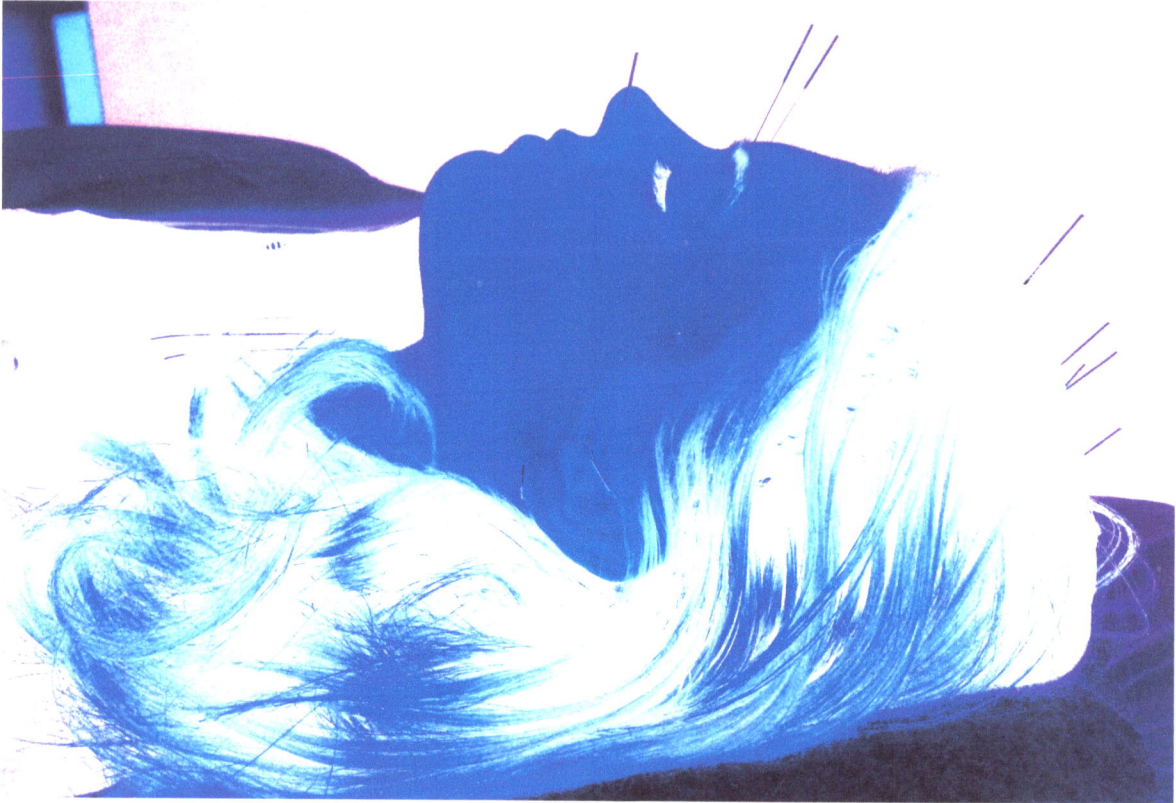

Picture 37. Acupuncture for stress reduction. Courtesy Joley.

Acupuncture, a practice that embodies precision and care, involves the insertion of thin, sterile needles into specific entry points. These points, which mark the anatomical and electromagnetic gateways into energy channels, are designed to allow the needle to glide into your body at the point of lowest electrical resistance. This meticulous approach and the practitioner's expertise ensure that acupuncture needles cause little or no pain, prioritizing your comfort and safety during the procedure.

The entry points are the gateways between your body's interior and external environments. The energy channel crosses the skin barrier and connects the inside with the outside of the body at the special small areas known as acupuncture points. The body's entry points, equipped with exceptional sensors that connect them directly to the heart and brain, are evidence of the fantastic aspects of your body's design. Their complex structure and precise functionality underscore the body's innate ability to heal and regulate itself.

Acupuncture intervention is excellent in accelerating or slowing down the functions of your body. If your body is distressed, acupuncture will reduce the intensity of the stress response and calm the information and energy flow.

Nerves, blood, and their cells, bodily fluids like the lymphatic fluid with water, minerals, and small molecules such as Oxygen (O2), Nitric Oxide NO, biochemical mediators, and hormones are the carriers of the initiated vitality movement.

If you have not yet experienced acupuncture, try it. You may be pleasantly surprised by how much medical acupuncture can reduce your stress and transform your distress into a sense of well-being in just 30 minutes. Approach it with an open mind and a sense of curiosity, and you may find a new avenue for healing and stress relief.

15

New way of your heartfelt life

"Forget the former things; do not dwell on the past. See, I am doing a new thing! Isaiah Chapter 43, Verse 18-19.

Boarding on your new lifestyle, the practice of abdominal orbital breathing is a journey of discovery. It connects you with the solar and pelvic plexus and your own Universe. As you delve into your respiratory muscle training, you will uncover a fascinating parallel. Just as our planet Earth has an orbit, so does your body. During inhalation, the energy of your breath follows a path from your crotch, alongside your spine, to the top of your head and then descending to your upper lip. During exhalation, visualize your breath energy traveling from your bottom lip to the crotch.

The revelation of the microcosmic orbit is truly transformative. Aligning your breath with your microcosmic orbit will not only enhance your brain energy channel but also elevate your vital energy to a higher level. This transformation may sometimes manifest as an emotional release. The tingling of your hand, legs, and sometimes the entire body, like under an energy shower, will inspire and motivate your soul and spirit.

In your mind, orbital breathing gets a new grid and representation. Remember that your breath not only moves invisible energy but also accelerates cerebrospinal fluid movements. This is your breath, a nurturing force that nourishes your brain and spine and cares for your overall well-being.

Be assertive and make some critical decisions in your new lifestyle. For example, start something new, like meditation or singing of the healing sounds.

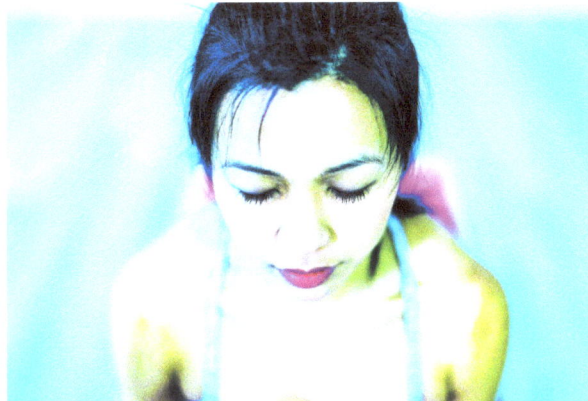

Picture 38. A young woman is engaged in meditation with her eyes closed. By Jussie2024. Own work. Wikipedia.

Meditation is a perfect time to refine your new orbital breathing. It can wipe away the amounting stress and bring inner peace. See how you can easily learn to practice meditation whenever needed. Spending even a few minutes meditating can help restore your calm and inner peace.

Singing specific sounds offers a holistic approach to healing and recovery. It addresses physical, emotional, and intellectual well-being. Sound therapy is a valuable tool for you. If you seek to overcome challenges and achieve a higher level of wellness by promoting relaxation, reducing stress, and encouraging emotional release, please try the healing sounds.

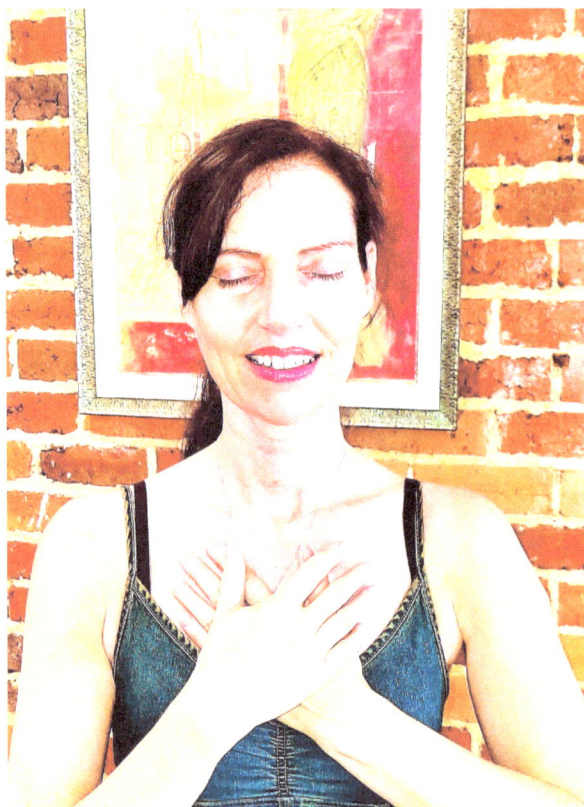

Picture39, Singing of the healing sound for the heart.

Courtesy Lindsay.

The healing sounds

The healing sound for the heart.

The sound 'A' is pronounced like in the word "Angel", for the heart's origin in the middle chest. You actively participate in your healing by gently laying your hands on your chest and feeling the heart vibrating with your sound.

The healing sound for the brain, mouth, teeth, and throat.

The sound "M," pronounced like in the word " Maria," is for the brain, the upper airways, neck, throat, teeth, and mouth. Please place your hands on your neck or on your face, repeat the sound several times, and perceive the vibrations of this region.

The healing sound for the liver.

The sound 'E' is pronounced like in the word "Emanuel." It is the healing sound for the liver. It is formed in the upper tummy on the right-hand side, where the liver and the gallbladder dwell. While singing the "E" sound, place your hands there to feel the vibrating liver.

The healing sound for the spleen and stomach.

The sound 'A,' pronounced like the word "Father," for spleen and stomach, is formed in the stomach and spleen region slightly on the left side of your tummy. While singing, place your hands there and repeat it until you feel this region will be moved gently.

The healing sound for the lungs.

The sound ' O', pronounced like in the word " Lord," for lungs, will resonate in the upper chest region. Place your hands on both sides of your collarbones. You will feel your lungs vibrating!

The healing sound for kidneys.

The sound "U," pronounced like in the word "You," is a healing sound for the kidneys and urinary bladder. Place your hands in the lower back region and feel the vibrations there.

Repetition is key to be effective. Sing each sound several times to fully experience the healing power of these sounds.

Your awareness of your body's wholeness and the new feeling of energy channels crossing through your body are joyful parts of this training. This new feeling of energy channels building an entire network in your body is a quantum experience and an amazing feeling of your re-energized body. Where attention goes, energy flows.

Opting out of hormone replacement therapy (HRT) can be highly beneficial. If you experience symptoms like hot flashes, consider a proven herbal formulation that works wonders: a blend of lady's mantle, yarrow, and horsetail. When prepared as a tisane (herbal infusion), this combination can provide significant relief and enhance your well-being.

Embrace the Hollywood Diet—a powerful lifestyle choice for a very efficient and pleasant detox. This entirely liquid diet is backed by effectiveness. It includes fresh-pressed pineapple juice, a variety of teas, coffee, mineral water, and fennel soup. Developed in the 1960s by Jane Fonda, it is a trusted method to detox, maintain satisfaction without hunger, and feel rejuvenated.

An interesting story about the Hollywood diet and why it was so popular is that you are not hungry even after several days, and your breath smells good. When you do not eat, your body will use an energy reserve to function—this is when you burn fat. Burning fat involves the release of ketone, which produces a foul smell. This unpleasant scent is usually released from the body through our breath, but not while you are on the Hollywood diet.

Perform your training and stretch your body daily. Discover energy channel training, a straightforward yet impactful approach to hormonal balance. Just 20 minutes of daily practice, whether through spinal flow, training of your energy channels, or yoga, can transform your health and boost your vitality remarkably. You can find more in the first book of my series, Medical Knowledge Made Easy. The book Grace in Movement, published in 2024, will improve your understanding of your health and bodily performance.

Experience the benefits of acupuncture and reflexology, two of the most effective methods for restoring hormonal balance. These techniques stimulate specific entry points along the energy channels in your body, help regulate hormone levels, and correct symptoms of imbalance. These safe, natural, and proven treatments can enhance your hormonal health.

Embrace your heart, your best friend. Your heart's role in maintaining the body's overall health is unparalleled. Skillfully re-balancing turbulent vortex flow and the swirling motion of blood caused by a temporarily rigid heart wall is paramount to its perfection.

It is masterful at preventing premature ventricular beats, ensuring smooth and uninterrupted blood flow. Your heart maintains a steady rhythm, gently pulsating throughout your body. With astounding endurance, it generates a regular heartbeat without fail for an average lifespan of about 100 or more years. Each heartbeat produces an electrical-evoked potential in your brain, running through the spine and nervous system to every corner of your body. This constant stream of information reaches your cells, activating their sensors and ultimately influencing your DNA.

But your heart is more than just a physical organ; it is a gateway to your emotions. It houses a large amount of messenger RNA (mRNA) molecules that stimulate the production of hormones related to your feelings. These hormones, such as oxytocin and dopamine, are essential in regulating the intensity of your emotional responses. The dynamic flow of information is a vibrant cascade of living signals. It renews itself with each heartbeat. Acknowledge the incredible power of your heart. It is not only essential for your survival but is also intimately connected to your emotional well-being. Listen to your heart and cherish every one of its heartbeats.

Thanks and gratitude

My heart goes to my wife, Angela. The MH17 disaster on 17 07 2014 was an epic challenge and extreme distress in our lives.

Our daughter Fatima Dyczynski (25), an Aerospace Engineer and a promising scientist in Airspace Systems Engineering, was on board of the civilian airliner Boeing 777, shot down in the most secret, covert operation of the Russian military along with 297 other passengers and crew, including 80 children.

Yet, Angela found the inner strength to call for scientific investigation in all our interviews with CNN, BBC, Canadian Broadcasting Corporation (CBC), and other TV and Media outlets worldwide. Angela used to say, "We need the science and criminal investigation, not condolences."

We promised our daughter during our first sleepless night after the MH17 disaster to search for her and go to the crash site. We went to Donetsk, a 12,000-km long way to the East of Ukraine. We visited the crash site of the Malaysian Flight MH17 to search for our daughter. We had to face war in an unprecedented way.

We went to East Ukraine two weeks after the MH17 disaster. We faced the emergency situation in Dnipropetrovsk (Dnipro) and the war in Donetsk. We walked the sunflower fields, filled with hope, hoping to find Fatima at the crash site.

Angela, when facing at the military checkpoints the young, well-trained, and masked Russian soldiers directing their guns against our bodies, the Canadian TV crew used to say to them, "Make love, not war." She spoke in Italian, which sounds like it is not from this world in these moments—*Fate l'amore, non la guerra*—while lifting her leg and showing them the high heels of her Italian shoes. It made them smile and let us through the military checkpoints.

Fatima's pioneering project for her Xoterra space high-tech start-up company was truly visionary. Her goal was to launch a constellation of 88 small satellites into low earth orbit (LEO). This space system engineering would have revolutionized Earth observation. Her vision was to make real-time Earth observation images accessible to everyone with a mobile phone, anytime, anywhere.

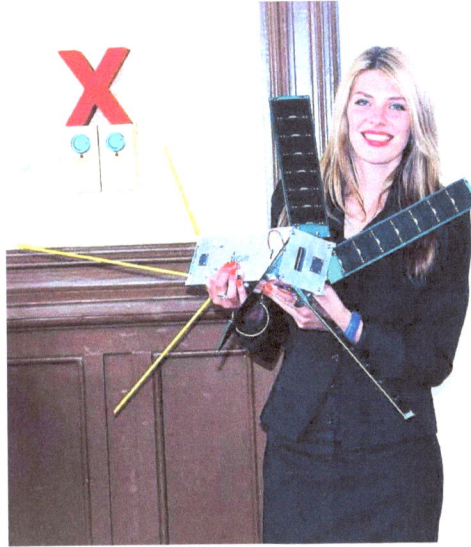

Fatima with a nanosatellite.

Let's make space personal: Fatima Dyczynski at TEDxGroningen

https://www.youtube.com/watch?v=VEbLvhRLwPo

This technology is a reality today, with companies like Space X using thousands of 'minisatellites.' Still, their weight is as much as a small car. With her untimely departure, the world lost a potential game-changer in the space industry.

I would like to thank my patients and my cardiology teachers equally. I am grateful for their contribution to the growth of my knowledge and experience about the heart and holistic Cardiology.

I am deeply indebted to Prof. Zdzisława Kornacewicz-Jach, a leading Cardiologist at the Medical University of Pomerania. Her influence has been profound, inspiring my interest in Cardiology for women. Her legacy as the great Lady of Polish cardiology will continue to inspire generations.

I extend my heartfelt thanks to Dr. Mary, a seasoned holistic GP with over 20 years of experience in metabolic stress management. Her profound insights on this topic have significantly enriched my understanding. I am honored to integrate her perspectives into this book.

Metabolic stress is the imbalance in your body caused by long-lasting cardiovascular stress and by low oxygenation of your body or lack of oxygen in the cells. Metabolic stress can also result from abnormal nutrient utilization and medication metabolism. It can be caused by deficiency or excess nutrients. It needs special attention. More often, metabolic stress is a response to low energy levels that can occur when your body's energy system is imbalanced, leading to disruptions in the metabolic wheel.

Metabolic stress disrupts your normal balance, causing a nutrient scarce. Nutrient scarcity can also cause inflammation and tissue damage. The principal manifestation of your nutrient scarcity is a chronic lack of energy, sometimes coined as chronic fatigue syndrome. Understanding metabolic stress can inspire you to take proactive steps to manage and mitigate your levels of Homocysteine, Vitamin B12, and Folate.

Metabolic stress occurs when your body needs more energy than it currently has. It can be caused by extreme emotional stress or strenuous exercises, such as high-intensity interval training or marathon running. It can also be a long-lasting intellectual effort, like studying for exams or working on a complex project. Your extraordinary energy expenses lead to a buildup of metabolites like lactate, phosphate, and hydrogen ions in the cerebrospinal fluid, brain and spine, heart muscle, and muscle cells.

Homocysteine, an indicator of metabolic stress, plays a significant role in heart health. It can be measured in the blood. Homocysteine is an amino acid your body can not completely process in distress. It indicates metabolic stress very clearly. It is also an indirect indicator of B12 vitamin deficiency and, eventually, Folate.

Specifically, when the heart is distressed, and a high level of Homocysteine is detected, it could contribute to blood clots and the increased risk of developing vulnerable plaques. It can indicate an additional risk to that of the 'bad cholesterol' inside your coronary arteries. The discovery of high Homocysteine levels can help guide the prevention and treatment of your heart in distress and manage metabolic stress for the good of heart health.

Also, I would like to express my deep gratitude to the beautiful pharmacist Yeena for her innovative nutriceutical, natural formulation similar to Statin. Yeena's work was inspired by my mention in the previous book, "Positive Heart Remodeling," about the benefits of red yeast rice for the heart and cardiovascular system.
She took this impulse and added her unique perspective, creating what I consider a Megacapsule. This formulation has proven to be a natural game-changer, normalizing the lipid profile and having a strong anti-inflammatory effect. It reduces stress in the cardiovascular system and metabolic stress as well. It helps to cool down the vulnerable plaques in the coronary arteries and supports positive heart remodeling.

Dr Jerzy George Dyczynski, MD, MBA, is a highly skilled physician and a seasoned Cardiologist with a strong interest in modern, conventional, and traditional medicine. His career as a medical doctor began in 1976 in Poland's emergency unit of a Cardiology Department. He has since demonstrated his adaptability and global perspective by working in various healthcare settings across Germany, Switzerland, China, and Australia, providing a diverse and comprehensive understanding of international medical practices.

Dr Jerzy holds a doctorate in Cardiology, a field in which he has made significant contributions through numerous books. He also recently initiated the Medical Knowledge Made Easy series in 2024, a series aimed at simplifying the medical language and guiding aid through complex healthcare systems. It is designed to encourage and foster everyone to be active, knowledgeable, and an expert on one's own health.

Dr George is deeply passionate about holistic medicine, particularly holistic heart health. He finds great joy in helping patients improve their wellness and well-being. With a clinical background as a medical doctor, specialist in internal medicine, and Cardiologist, he is well-equipped to address a wide range of complex conditions, including cardiovascular and stress-related issues.

From 2008 to 2009, Dr George worked as a researcher in Heart-Brain Medicine and as a clinical acupuncturist for outpatients at Edith Cowan University Clinic in Perth. His dedication to a holistic approach is a cornerstone of his professional and personal life, reflecting his unwavering commitment to patient care. His extensive training in energy channels, traditional gymnastics for health, and over 30 years of kung fu martial arts practice demonstrates his open-mindedness and desire to inspire others to explore holistic health.

His most recent works include "*The Dyczynski Program: Healing the Intelligent Heart,*" published in 2022, and the series Medical Knowledge Made Easy, the first book, "*Grace in Movement,*" and the second, "*Positive Heart Remodeling.*" The third book of this series *is Your Healing Hands. The Power of Reflexology* was published at the end of 2024.

www.ingramcontent.com/pod-product-compliance
Lightning Source LLC
Chambersburg PA
CBHW050908210326
41597CB00002B/67